AMBULATORY HEALTH CARE

Case Studies for the Health Services Executive

Edited by

Austin Ross, MPH, and Mary Richardson, Ph.D.

Published by

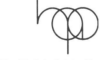

Health Administration Press
A Division of the Foundation of the American
College of Healthcare Executives

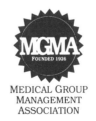

MEDICAL GROUP
MANAGEMENT
ASSOCIATION

00   99   98   97   96   5   4   3   2   1

Library of Congress Cataloging-in-Publication Data

Ambulatory health care case studies for the health services executive / edited by Austin Ross and Mary Richardson.

p.   cm.
Includes bibliographical references.
ISBN 1-56793-044-1
1. Hospitals — Outpatient services — Administration — Case studies.
2. Ambulatory medical care — Administration — Case studies. I. Ross, Austin.
II. Richardson, Mary, 1944– .
[DNLM: 1. Ambulatory Care — case studies. WB 101 A497 1996]
RA974.A44   1996
362.1'068—dc20
DNLM/DLC
for Library of Congress   96-12939
                                                                                    CIP

Copyright © Medical Group Management Association, 1996

Health Administration Press
A Division of the Foundation of the American College of
Healthcare Executives

MEDICAL GROUP
MANAGEMENT ASSOCIATION

One North Franklin Street, Suite 1700
Chicago, IL 60606-3491
(312) 424-2800

104 Inverness Terrace East
Englewood, CO 80112-5306
(303) 799-1111

Contents

Part I.   Introduction to the Use of Cases & This Book

Part II.   Health Services Background

Part III.   The Organization

System Organization and Integration

Organizational relationships between the physicians and staff at the Community Clinical Oncology Program at Oxford Medical Center, and between these physicians and the research community at large, are carefully explored. Clearly, the organizational complexity is creating problems for Dr. Smith and his colleagues. The accessing of patients for protocol studies is critical to the success of the research unit, and ways to resolve the organizational problems must be found in order to advance the cause of the research program.

Key Words: Research organization, affiliate relationships, physician referrals, community programs.

Decision Making and Leadership

Clinical and Managerial Quality Improvement

Management of Human Resources

Part IV. Practice Management

Group Practice Management and Administration

A physician group practice, one of two in a midsize city, is facing financial difficulties because of a recent expansion in primary care satellite clinics and the changing health care reimbursement structure. The clinic manager must address the potential effect on physician income and the need to reduce expenses, including reducing staff positions. Dealing with three points in time, the case offers a perspective on the cumulative decisions to be made.

Key Words: Physician group practice, cost management, downsizing, continuous quality improvement.

Mergers and Acquisitions

In a two-hospital community, pressure begins to build to bring the hospitals closer together to reduce costs. One hospital is from a Catholic system, and the other has a community ownership base. Logic would suggest that duplication in this 80,000-citizen community is expensive. The two hospitals employ a consulting team to facilitate the study process. Medical staff and other issues complicate the decision-making process.

Key Words: Merger/affiliation, acquisition, culture conflict, mission and values.

A primary care practice seeks to form an integrated primary care network by merging with a larger system. The author focuses on strategic planning methods used to identify strategic vision, goals for group and individual practitioners, and key decision criteria, and how to deal with physician loss of control. The case documents the process of selecting a partner, including the use of force-field analysis.

Key Words: Physician group practice, strategic planning, merger/affiliation, dealing with change, physician loss of control.

Managed Care

Planning and Strategy

Part V. Short Interactive Case Studies

Although the cases in this book may be based in part on factual situations or include approaches to problem solving that were actually used, they refer to fictional entities and characters.

Foreword

*We must welcome the future, remembering that soon it will be the
past. And we must respect the past, remembering that once it was all
that was humanly possible.*
— George Santayana

The genesis for this book is related to the case study tradition advanced by the
Harvard School of Business Administration. In 1962, the Medical Group Management Association sponsored a program at Harvard for which a set of specific
case studies was prepared. While time has taken its toll on the relevancy of
those cases, the need for a new work transcending this early experience has
been often noted. We now have that work for at least three reasons worth noting as we look to the future.

First, there is the changing nature of environmental forces shaping health
care services organization and delivery. A relatively stable environment in the
early 1960s meant that most factors affecting business decision making were
found within an organization's walls. Today it is more often factors outside an
organization's walls that drives decision making. Furthermore, as we focus on
clinical decision-making processes, organizations' walls become barriers that
give way to management processes encompassing both clinical and business
interests.

Second, there are changes in academia relevant to the education of health
services executives. In brief, early academic leadership came from notable hospital executives bringing their case experience to campuses in search of
intellectual stimulation, legitimacy, and a new venue for mentoring The pen-
dulum then swung toward faculty coming from various academic disciplines.
Field work, including case studies from a variety of health care settings, provided an opportunity for theories to be supported or questioned. We are now
realizing the power of teaming in which practitioners and faculty both respect-
fully encompass experience and theory by working side by side to improve
our learning processes continuously.

1

Third, there is the changing role of professional associations. In the past, the value of opportunities for networking has ranked very high on the list of reasons why people join professional associations. Is not "networking" at some operational level the same as "real-time case studies"? And, as this activity goes both on-line in cyberspace and more face-to-face at the local level, what will be the future role of professional associations in networking?

So it is around the theme of integration that a diverse team of authors, with collaborative support of the American College of Healthcare Executives and the Medical Group Management Association, developed the following cases for use in various settings. The great majority of us who were directly involved in this project would not know one another if we passed on the street today. Collectively, however, there is satisfaction in knowing we did today what is humanly possible to help advance the state of practice — and knowing either as preparers or users of this work, there is an excellent chance we will be working together in the future.

Fred Graham, Ph.D., FACMPE, CAE
Senior Vice President, Chief Operating Officer
Medical Group Management Association
February 14, 1996

Preface

by Austin Ross and Mary Richardson

We approached this task with considerable trepidation. There are a number of excellent case study books in use, and case studies have a way of becoming quickly outdated when the health care industry is undergoing such change. If federal legislation comes out of the starting gate, it may shorten the life of case studies even more.

But on reflection it became apparent that in a volatile arena some risks have to be taken, and that it is very useful to have cases that portray a system in change. Cases locked in a traditional approach are no longer applicable.

Having made that decision, we elected to proceed. And with the encouragement of Fred Graham of the Medical Group Management Association and Daphne Grew of Health Administration Press, we decided to devote our energies toward collecting a variety of cases that cover the range of ambulatory care, but to focus on cases that contribute to an understanding of the development of integrated delivery systems.

We also wanted to do something that was even more challenging. We wanted to compile cases that could be used not only in the academic setting with health administration students, but in the practice setting by busy clinic and system executives engaged in comprehensive team-building processes.

As a result, we elected to build on cases that provide different levels of activity for students and practitioners. At the core are a handful of cases intended to require strategic and analytical thought. These cases provide a rich mixture of facts and are structured to challenge complex decision-making processes.

For supporting players, we identified a number of cases that may require less in-depth analysis, but that are time limited and reflect the state of the art of decision making—where all the facts may not come easily to hand but managerial and executive decisions are required.

And then finally, we selected a number of quick, highly interactive case studies that can be used as tools to sharpen on-line encounters. These are intended to test and build the skills of the participants, emphasizing role playing. We have found these latter cases of considerable value because they provide special opportunities for students and others to display their newly acquired classroom skills in a way that reinforces the learning process.

It will be up to the reader to determine whether we have met these rather ambitious goals.

Acknowledgments

We are indebted to Fred Graham of Medical Group Management Association, who provided the initial incentive when he called one evening and suggested that it was about time to produce a case book focusing on the ambulatory care world, and to Daphne Grew of Health Administration Press, who agreed to enter into a joint venture with MGMA in the publishing of the book.

The willingness of those who contributed the case material was outstanding and gratifying. Case authors produced quality material on time, which immensely eased the editors' task.

We also wish to acknowledge our deep gratitude to Nancy Moncreiff from Health Administration Press, who headed the editing process, and to Barbara Hamilton from MGMA who so effectively advised us along the trail. Refining a text that had so many contributors was a significant undertaking.

Finally, we wish to acknowledge particularly the contributions of Donna Jones from the Department of Health Services at the University of Washington, who made this project possible and in the process kept our feet to the fire by meeting those deadlines.

Austin Ross
Mary Richardson

PART I

Introduction to the Use of Cases and This Book

Conducting the Case Study

by Austin Ross

Case studies are not classroom time fillers. Including case studies just to round out an educational experience does an injustice to one of the most valuable teaching tools available to an instructor. Lecturing usually serves as the mainstay of a course. Through lecturing, the instructor disseminates information on the assumption that students will absorb it and get its point. The intelligent use of supplemental case studies advances the cause both by transmitting information and by more fully engaging students in the process of learning. Further, the case study provides the instructor with critical feedback as to how well students are synthesizing information.

In class, the quiet or disengaged student holds back; the articulate and confident student shines. The practice world is similar. The boss talks, and the employee listens. Vivacious employees participate actively; quiet ones may be overlooked. Case studies help bring quiet students or employees out from the wings and onto the stage. But this does not happen by accident. Instructors not only have to know their students' strengths and weaknesses but must be willing to invest time crafting the case study experience to meet their needs. This is an important point because, to carry off a good case study in the classroom, the instructor needs to be several steps ahead of the students. A problem arises when the instructor lacks an experience base (for example, in ambulatory care). A lack of knowledge about the details of a case may push instructors into selecting conceptually broader and safer cases and discourage them from seeking out the cases that might be of most value to the students. Instructors who feel they lack hands-on experience may opt to use older and safer cases.

This book of cases, with a focus on ambulatory care, is intended to offer some variety to the instructor's teaching tools, whether that instructor is based in the academic setting or in the practice world.

Case Variety

The quality of case studies is variable, and there is a paucity of good cases dealing with ambulatory care. Shortcomings in the existing inventory of cases in the ambulatory health care field relate to the perception — prevalent until recently — that ambulatory care is relatively unimportant in the scheme of health care delivery. For decades, case studies have focused on the delivery of care in hospitals in highly organized care units. There hasn't really been a mature market for ambulatory care case studies and, although the need for them is now clear, creating that needed inventory takes time.

One reason for this is that instructors in health administration programs tend to lack personal experience in group practice or ambulatory care, so those who could work up cases from an academic viewpoint are few in number. In past decades, there has been more excitement and attention involved in the development of case studies involving integrated systems and the major organizations. In addition, the funding for solid health services research has tended to focus on major policy issues rather than the management of a selected subcomponent of the system, such as managing a medical practice.

Suddenly, however, ambulatory care and other alternatives to inpatient care have arrived at center stage. Different questions are now being posed. How physicians are compensated, for example, surfaces as an issue in the determination of incentives to contain costs. Does the organizational structure in group practices affect how care is delivered? How does a manager learn about the complexities of executing or initiating change in a physician-dominated environment? The list of seemingly new issues is endless, and there will be a lag in time before a number of good cases surface that are designed to demonstrate clearly and cleanly the organizational principles involved in differentiating the management issues of ambulatory care from the more traditional organizational approaches.

Another complicating factor is the diversity of definitions of ambulatory care. The hospital as an organizational unit is relatively cleanly defined. Group practice is definable, but organizational settings range from the private group through public health agencies and beyond. Integrated health care delivery systems further confuse the picture because (properly) health care represents a continuum of practices, not just ambulatory care any more than just hospitals or integrated delivery systems.

So this book represents a modest effort to add to the inventory of cases targeted at aspects of ambulatory care. The reader will quickly note that, while there is an emphasis on the ambulatory side, some of the cases in this book brush up against other components of the system — including the critical aspect of policy development.

Source of Cases

The source of a number of these cases is noteworthy. We turned to a small number of academic leaders to set the pace. Their input and authorship of several key cases were important. To develop the majority of cases, we called on individuals working in the ambulatory practice setting. In addition, following Jim Hepner's trail of compiling cases from practitioners in the hospital field who were preparing material needed for advancement to Fellowship in the American College of Healthcare Executives, we approached those aspiring to advancement in the American College of Medical Practice Executives (previously known as the American College of Medical Group Administrators). They proved a rich source of case study material.

Case Criteria

In pulling the cases together, we watched for cases that met four primary criteria:

1. *Timeliness*. We sought cases that focus on current management issues. Universities properly examine concepts and theory. The learning experience can be enriched by cases that are practice-oriented and up-to-the-moment in content. In days past, it was possible to rely on a handful of classical case studies that displayed clearly defined organization or theoretical objectives. The setting and the environment were perhaps less important than the classical features of the cases themselves. This doesn't work as well today because of the massive changes taking place in the field. The state of the internal and external environment affects decision making more than ever. Thus the settings for the cases are very current.

2. *Unit scale*. We also attempted to find cases that represent different scales of operation, ranging all the way from the small single-specialty group practice to the larger integrated organization. We were particularly sensitive to the needs of managers in smaller operating units, who frequently have to flounder their way through the maze without having at hand the levels of expertise found in larger units. It is not sufficient for students graduating these days to know just why something is occurring; they need to get quickly into the how-to side of the equation. A number of the cases in this book contain information on how to do it.

3. *Practical application*. We placed a premium on finding real situations. In a number of the cases, the authors carefully spell out their solutions to the defined problems. The challenge to students and instructors alike will be to second-guess some of those solutions. Identifying the logic the authors used in arriving at their positions should provide some intriguing teaching opportunities.

4. *Applicability in both academic and practice settings.* Downsizing and the very real needs of the health care industry to reduce costs are unquestionably affecting organizations' ability to invest in management training. Investment in training is often one of the first functions weakened. Smaller organizations that rely on sending representatives to meetings to upgrade their competencies find new budgets restricting their ability to do so. Employers now have a greater expectation that newly hired staff come equipped to function as decision makers. They expect managers to arrive with the necessary tools and may be unable to invest in continuing education. Case studies can help accelerate skill learning, and we looked for cases that blur the differences between the classroom and the practice world.

Case Objectives

The instructor who draws from the inventory of cases in this book will find that a number of them, representing very real situations, cross organizational and technical boundaries. For the most part, however, the cases are loosely drawn and not academically cited or tied to clearly defined theoretical concepts. This then represents a challenge for the instructor. To use the cases successfully, the instructor must carefully determine in advance how to integrate them into the curriculum. The cases are building blocks; the instructor must decide how to build the pier.

Because cases may be used to accomplish a variety of objectives, instructors must make clear decisions concerning the goals of case study exercises. A case study approach also requires an adequate system of evaluation and feedback so that concurrent course adjustments can be made.

Cases can be chosen to further multiple ends. For example, cases can (1) build skills and competencies, (2) disseminate information, (3) measure the absorption of information by students, (4) provide live performance feedback to participants and instructors, and (5) strengthen instructor competency. Instructors obviously determine the objective and build the theater in which the case is used.

For those teaching analytical approaches, case studies based on substantive data are essential. Instructors looking for that dimension in this book will be disappointed; such case studies are still hard to find.

For those seeking cases in decision making, leadership development and strategic planning, the offerings are more complete. The book includes cases that lend themselves to issues of conflict resolution and negotiation, with leadership development a fairly common thread. And, as noted earlier, a number of cases lend themselves to second-guessing the case writers' decisions. Opportunities abound for changing the case outcome in class through changing key facts during the process of analyzing the case.

Categories of Cases

Generally cases can be classified into two categories: those designed to enhance individual expertise and those designed to strengthen oral interactive skills and team involvement.

Of course, no case is limited to a single category. Both categories are applicable. How a case is introduced and applied determines which one predominates.

Cases also can be assigned well in advance or sprung on students, depending again on the learning objective. Dropping a case on a class adds a component of excitement and reality that isn't there when students have that week or so to prepare in advance. Real life demands that some cases be used without advance notice. Group exercises without advance notice are useful to the instructor who is interested in helping students develop that crucial ability to think on their feet.

The rigor of how the case is applied is important. The instructor has to be ahead of the students and capable of conducting a live exercise. Students will know whether the instructor is tuned into the process or is escaping from the necessary rigors associated with the well-presented case study.

Guidelines and Conduct of Case Studies

This section is directed at the instructor and is basic in content. The reader needs to remember that the audience of this case book is not solely the well-trained educator but also the vulnerable manager on the front line who may be working with a shortfall of resources while developing new management teams. Readers who are experienced in conducting case studies may wish to skip this section.

Selecting the Case

To maximize the learning experience, the instructor must draw the right case study from the quiver. The teaching objective drives the process. Using a case study without clearly deciding in advance what is to be accomplished would be sloppy teaching. Objectives may be short- or long-range, but the case study should relate to the teaching syllabus and the curriculum.

When it is time to select a case, the instructor must consider the dynamics of its presentation. What information has been provided students that suggests the case process might add to their knowledge base? Would it be helpful now to provide students with opportunities to address questions as individuals, polishing their personal assessment techniques, or are they ready for a group dynamics approach? Tailoring the case study to the educational needs of the moment is the crux of the matter. The instructor needs to anticipate the effect of the case study on the class or group. What exactly will its use contribute to the cause of learning? If instructors come up short in answering this question, they might give second thoughts to using the case.

Testing It in Action

Case studies do not arrive on the scene fully developed and well executed. Instructors may need to present a case several times to flush out into the open its full subtleties. Instructors need to be patient with the process, learning from each presentation and modifying the approach, always keeping in mind that the dynamics of the class are changing, too. No two classes are identical. Students and managers bring with them different skills and backgrounds, and the instructor's task is vastly complicated by this diversity of talent. Is it any wonder that instructors opt for lectures over case studies? Constant assessment and refinement, however, pay off. The flexibility of the case study sharpens instructional skills and adds to the liberation of thought for both students and instructor.

Presenting the Case

Other aspects of case presentation are obvious. Always provide clear front-end instructions. Take time not only to describe the case process but also to share with the class or group the learning objectives of the case. Why keep them a secret?

Maintain control of the process. The group-process case that develops well does not always end up as planned. The instructor must at times intervene to help maintain a reasonable course. But instructors are also cautioned to allow latitude, since unforeseen turns can be great contributors to the pursuit of knowledge.

Look for opportunities to stretch thinking. Cases prepared in writing by an individual and those that follow a group dynamic process are both enhanced when the instructor is capable of taking an observation and moving the thought to a new level. The instructor accomplishes this most commonly through the appropriate use of the right question.

There are also certain aspects of classroom hygiene that should be maintained. For example, embarrassing a student may sharpen that student's response time the next time around or satisfy the ego of a control-minded instructor, but tactics that embarrass the student or the group are destructive to the case study process. A high intellectual and personal tone is mandatory.

Instructors also need to require students to consider issues of confidentiality. Case studies take on a life of their own when students use facts of local health care events in determining answers. Students need to know that confidentiality is essential to the discussion. Instructors should deal positively with lapses in confidentiality. Trust is an important element in the classroom.

With every case presentation, the instructor should look for feedback. Much of the feedback is informal. An alert instructor senses when things are or are not going well. Formal periodic feedback from the students is also crucial, such as written, confidential, end-of-the-quarter evaluations. When evaluating cases, the instructor should focus on their applicability to the objectives of the course.

A final word of advice to the instructor is to develop and apply listening skills. An instructor who continually interrupts the case process through overinvolvement affects it negatively.

While much of this advice pertains to group or team-building exercises, the same principles apply to the case study given as an individual assignment. Clear projection of the objective, follow-through on the evaluation, and respect for the hygiene of the process are all important to a successful outcome.

Expectations

Students should be able to count on five facts. (1) The instructor is prepared and in control and knows where the case is headed. (2) The rules of the case are determined in advance. (3) The case contributes to the knowledge base. (4) The instructor is trustful and nonjudgmental. (5) Personal risks to the students are minimized.

In turn, the instructor should be able to expect that students are: (1) rigorous in preparation, (2) willing to be courageous and take chances, (3) respectful of confidences, and (4) demanding in expecting teaching excellence from the instructor.

Summary

Properly used, case studies add great value to the classroom. This book provides new cases to enrich the educational processes of those intending to pursue practice in the ambulatory field. The additional dividend is that using these cases in the right setting may broaden the instructor's competency in teaching ambulatory care.

Using and Analyzing Case Studies

by Mary Richardson

By describing real situations or problems to illustrate key concepts, case studies help instructors integrate practice with theory. A case study, to some degree, brings the practice setting into the classroom. Through case analysis and problem solving, students can demonstrate how well they understand theories and concepts presented in the classroom by applying them to real-world situations. Thus, the case experience can elevate the teaching process from lecture to interaction.

To use a case effectively, instructors must

1. As part of their own preparation, clearly identify the teaching point or purpose of a case
2. Engage the students in thinking creatively about case analysis and problem solving
3. Identify approaches to be used for effective case analysis
4. Make clear to students that there may be no single or correct answer
5. Communicate to the students the criteria upon which their case analysis will be evaluated

For their part, students must

1. Recognize case situations will not necessarily present all the information necessary for problem solving or promote simple or even single solutions
2. Be willing to inject themselves into the case and to be creative in their approach to problem identification and analysis

3. Identify the assumptions they make and the logic upon which they base their case analysis

4. Be able to articulate their analysis effectively orally or in writing or both

Generally, there are three steps in case analysis: summarizing the facts, inferring information from facts, and identifying the problems and implementing the solutions.

Summarizing the facts. By systematically summarizing the facts of a case, one can identify the framework within which it is presented, to determine areas in which there are gaps or irregularities in information. If the case is being analyzed by a group, students may discover they hold different perspectives or views of the facts.

Inferring information from facts. Who are the principal players in the case, and what are their perspectives? How are the players interrelated, and how do their relationships affect the case? What are the critical issues as defined by key players, and how does the relative influence of the players alter or affect the importance of these issues? What are the key organizations or groups involved? To what extent must one consider individual perspectives versus organizational or group responses to the issues presented?

Identifying the problems and implementing solutions. What problems does the case raise? Are they obvious, or are some more subtle than others? Why do they exist? Who will need to be involved in addressing them? Where will support come from? Resistance? What information, technology, or other resources are needed to address these problems? To what extent are the problems systems problems, which lend themselves to structural changes, and to what extent are they people problems, which may need to be addressed by changing individual attitudes and behavior? Is the time frame important? That is to say, should there be short-term or interim solutions, or long-term solutions, or both?

A Primer on How to Use This Casebook

by Austin Ross

First, determine your teaching objective. Then review the casebook's table of contents, which contains a brief description of each case and its "key words" to help you identify its contents.

After selecting a case, focus on the questions at the end and modify them to meet your teaching objectives. Design how and when to use the case. Thought should be given as to how much classroom time should be allowed for case presentation and discussion. Presenting a case without adequate discussion time is detrimental to the learning process.

In all cases the instructor should define expectations. The options for case presentation are limitless. Cases could be assigned for advance reading and study or used on a highly "unrehearsed" interactive basis. For example, cases could be assigned with different teams of students taking different positions. The shorter interactive cases, assigned without advance notice, might meet the teaching objective of encouraging students to "think on their feet."

Practice contributes significantly to the quality of a case study presentation. It is suggested, with case study teaching, that a series of cases be used during the quarter to sharpen the students' skill base. The variety in case content needs to be considered carefully in order to meet teaching objectives.

When conducting case presentations with student teams, it may be useful to involve other students in assessing the presentation. Factors to be considered in such an assessment include:

- How clearly are facts and issues presented?
- Is there a clear understanding of any assumptions made as part of the analysis?
- Are case findings and conclusions consistent with the facts of the case?
- Does the presentation team clearly present and support conclusions?

PART II

Health Services Background

Health Care in the United States

by Mary Richardson

Health care in the United States had its beginnings in public health services, focused on communities, and aimed at preventing or reducing illness associated with infectious diseases. Health concerns were caused by epidemics of infectious diseases such as the plague, cholera, typhoid, smallpox, influenza, and yellow fever, particularly in heavily populated areas such as New York City. For example, a cholera epidemic in the middle 1800s resulted in the deaths of more than 5,000 people in New York City, while yellow fever killed 9,000 in New Orleans in 1853, another 2,500 in 1854 and 1855, and an additional 5,000 in 1858 (Torrens 1993). Hospital or other institutional care was limited to individuals whose illness was so serious it could not be treated in the home. It wasn't until this century that hospitals gained a dominant role in the delivery of health care services.

As public health efforts brought epidemics under control, however, attention shifted to the health and medical needs of the individual. The structure of health care today, with its emphasis on illness and medical care interventions delivered in an institutionally based service system, developed in the late 1800s and this century. The forces that combined to bring about that change included the development of a strong scientific basis for medical practice, enhanced physician and nurse training, a substantial increase in access to medical care services through the creation of insurance mechanisms, and the development of a hospital-based system of service delivery. Public health, with its roots in community wide surveillance and monitoring and its emphasis on preventing illness, now accounts for less than 3 percent of overall health care expenditures.

Developing the Medical Care System

The Scientific Base

At the turn of the century, the scientific method was being applied to the practice of medicine, and medical science began to influence the techniques and delivery of medical care. Alexander Fleming's discovery of penicillin in 1928 began an unprecedented era of advances in medical science and a revolution in care based on the availability of antibiotics. As infectious disease came under the control of antibiotics, the major cause of disease and death among Americans became chronic diseases such as heart disease, cancer, and stroke, accounting for two-thirds of all deaths by 1990 (ibid.). Arthritis, blindness, and arteriosclerosis have become the primary causes of disability.

Biomedical research, although heavily funded by the federal government, was undertaken by universities, thereby transforming education in medicine and nursing and placing it in the academic setting while promoting the expansion of new, specialized areas of health care practice. Prior to the advent of a scientific base in medicine, physician training varied greatly. Before 1900, a large number of small, poorly staffed, freestanding medical colleges existed throughout the country (ibid.). In 1910, Alexander Flexner published a study of medical education in the United States and Canada, commissioned by the Carnegie Foundation for the Advancement of Teaching. Based in part on Dr. Flexner's recommendations, smaller, poorly funded medical schools began to close, and larger, better- financed schools began to adopt more fully the advancing technology of medical science, and affiliated with universities. Physicians began to be trained as scientists and practitioners.

The advancement of medical science and the practice of medical care received a substantial boost in 1930 when the U.S. Public Health Service's Hygienic Laboratory was transformed into the National Institutes of Health, with broad authority for medical research. Medical science provided significant advancement in many areas, including the development of highly sophisticated, technologically based diagnostic and surgical techniques, and pharmaceutical interventions. In fact, the United States enters the twenty-first century with the most technologically sophisticated medical care system in the history of the world.

The Financial Base

Medical care in the United States was, for many years, considered an individual responsibility; people were generally expected to find their own physician or other care provider. Besides physicians, practitioners included nurses, midwives, and practitioners within ethnic communities such as curanderos within the Hispanic community and medicine men within Native American communities. Payment for services was the responsibility of the individual receiving the care, and the caregiver charged fees based on the specific services provided. When a person had limited means for payment, physicians often offered a sliding fee scale. Payment also took the form of bartering services or goods rather than the payment of cash. Communities assumed the financial responsibility of providing health care for some citizens, forming charitable institutions such as clinics and hospitals to provide health care for people who were indigent.

The concept of health insurance was not introduced in the United States until the 1920s. The first insurance plans were structured after European insurance approaches and were generally offered as a benefit of employment. Examples of early insurers were Blue Cross, organized to pay for hospital care, and later Blue Shield, which paid for physician care. Prepaid plans, which provide both medical care and insurance coverage for a set fee, were initiated during this same period but failed to increase in size in these early years because of substantial resistance from organized medicine. Insurance coverage has expanded to include other licensed providers, such as psychologists, over the years. However, coverage for services provided by nonphysician providers has remained limited in scope.

Health-related "social insurance," sponsored by the government, was introduced in 1914 with the passage of the first worker's compensation law. Payments were allowed for the replacement of wages lost due to disability and for some portion of the medical care required by the disability. Other government-supported health care consisted of federal funding for state-based public health initiatives and funding for special hospitals for merchant seaman, Native Americans, military personnel, and veterans. State payment for health care services was largely tied to the provision of public health services including indigent care, and medical care for persons who were incarcerated or who were institutionalized for chronic conditions and disabilities such as psychiatric disorders or mental retardation.

The federal government became far more involved in the provision of insurance in 1965 with the passage of Title XVIII of the Social Security Act (Medicare) aimed at assuring medical care for persons over the age of 65, and Title XIX (Medicaid) aimed at assuring medical care for poor persons. In order to participate in the Medicaid program, state governments must match federal funds and assume responsibility for administration. Medicare is administered at the federal level and does not require matching state funds.

Health insurance, and particularly the creation of Medicare and Medicaid, promoted access to health care for millions of Americans. It is estimated that, by the 1980s, health insurance covered approximately 76 percent of the population (Health Insurance Association of America 1986). During this same period of time, technological advances substantially improved the sophistication of health care services. Insurance coverage, with its emphasis on medical care, was quick to embrace new technologies and the growing specialization of medicine. Thus substantial numbers of people found themselves able to afford sophisticated medical care, including new technology as it developed.

The Institutional Base

Assisted by the advance of medical science and the development of insurance linked heavily to physician care, physicians evolved as the primary practitioners of medical care. Initially, physicians practiced independently, opening their own offices and delivering care in the office or in the patient's home. In the early days, care delivery did not demand a lot of technology, and physicians could carry with them most of what they needed. Rapidly expanding technology and medical specialization, however, changed the pattern of medical care practice. Physicians now practice in a variety of settings including solo practice, although such practice is declining, as physicians join together in both single- and multispecialty group practices. Physicians may base their practices in hospitals as independent practitioners with admitting privileges, or as salaried staff members. Rarely do physicians provide care in patients' homes, in part because the technology is no longer portable.

Hospitals as we know them today grew out of the almshouses or poorhouses that served the poor and homeless. People with infectious diseases, chronic conditions, and mental illnesses were all housed together in unsanitary and generally poor conditions (Haglund and Dowling 1993). Medical care was secondary to the primary function of housing indigent or mentally incompetent persons and isolating them from the other members of the community. During the latter part of the nineteenth century, however, medical departments or infirmaries broke away and became separate medical care institutions. Community hospitals began appearing in the late 1700s and early 1800s, in response to physicians' desire for facilities appropriate to the practice of obstetrics or surgery (ibid.). Pennsylvania Hospital in Philadelphia, established in 1751, was the first hospital, followed by hospitals in New York City, Boston, and New Haven, Connecticut.

Advances in medical technology, enhanced physician and nurse training, the advent of health insurance, and the entry of government financing all contributed toward a substantial growth in both the number and type of hospitals in the twentieth century. The Hill-Burton Hospital and Survey Construction Act in 1946 provided federal grants to communities so they could construct hospitals and other health facilities, thereby substantially increasing the number of hospital beds nationally, as well as increasing the relative number of hospitals in rural areas and small communities. In other instances, physicians built and owned hospitals. With the growth in the hospital industry, however, investor-owned organizations began forming for the purpose of buying, building, and managing hospitals, thus creating a new type of proprietary organization. Hospitals today include not-for-profit facilities owned by local communities, state and federal governments, and religious organizations, and proprietary facilities generally owned by groups of investors including physician groups.

Hospitals now range from short-stay hospitals, which provide acute, general medical care, to extended-stay institutions providing services for people with chronic conditions. The predominant type (accounting for 92 percent of the approximately 6,650 hospitals nationwide) and the most technologically sophisticated are short-stay hospitals in which patients remain less than 25 days.

Patients in long-stay hospitals include persons with physical conditions such as tuberculosis, those who are mentally ill, and those with cognitive disabilities such as mental retardation. Many early hospitals were created for and primarily serve people with a specific condition, such as tuberculosis or a chronic psychiatric condition. When people are hospitalized with chronic conditions and disabilities, cure is generally not the goal. Rather, restoration or promotion of function lost as a result of the condition, or prevention of further deterioration, are the goals. Persons with chronic conditions and disabilities often require a range of health and social services.

Another type of long-term care facility is the nursing home or skilled nursing facility, usually smaller than a hospital, serving 100 or fewer people. A nursing home may operate as a freestanding facility, a unit of a hospital, or a part of a retirement center. People who are unable to remain at home because of the severity of their chronic conditions or disability may be cared for in a nursing home. In fact, as public policy changes caused a reduction in hospitals serving persons who are mentally ill or mentally retarded, nursing homes became a substitute for the provision of long-term custodial care previously received in the larger institutional settings. Nursing home care, which increased by 22 percent between 1973 and 1985, is expected to continue to grow as the number of older adults increases as a percentage of the overall population. However, there is also a considerable trend to reduce utilization of nursing home care by creating alternative community- and home-based services.

Public policy over the last three decades has moved away from hospitalizing, or "institutionalizing" persons of all ages with chronic conditions or disabilities. These policy directions are the result, in part, of improved medical technology and better medical management of such conditions, making it possible for people to live more independent lives in a community setting. Psychotropic medications, for example, make it possible for many persons with severe psychiatric conditions to stabilize their condition and live independently or with their families. In addition, professionals and policymakers, led by consumer advocates, came to understand that long-term hospitalization or lengthy nursing home stays were unnecessary for many people previously committed without recourse or the availability of alternative community-based services. In fact, in many instances such institutionalization was shown to result in deteriorating physical and cognitive function. Thus, there has been a substantial move away from the use of such hospitals, accompanied by an increase in community-based alternatives.

Toward Systems Integration

Largely because of expanded access, and increased specialization and sophistication of medical practice, health care costs have grown faster than the overall economy for nearly 30 years . Health care as a percentage of the gross national product rose from 5.3 percent in 1960 to nearly 14 percent in 1994 (Sonnefeld et al. 1991). Rising health care costs are reflected in increasing insurance rates which in turn affect employers, who generally provide health insurance as an employee benefit; and state and federal governments, which fund insurance for adults over the age of 65, persons with disabilities, and poor people. The rising costs of medical care and insurance are now contributing to a decline in the proportion of Americans who have health insurance. Growing concern over those without financial access to health care prompted research by the National Center for Health Statistics, which estimated that in 1989 approximately 34 million Americans, or 15 percent of the population, fell into this category. This included unprecedented numbers of persons who were employed, but did not receive insurance as a condition of their employment, and their dependents.

Concern over increased costs of health care prompted the federal government to attempt a variety of regulatory controls. Generally, these controls have been aimed at managing the costs of hospital and physician services through rate-setting efforts. In the early 1980s, Medicare introduced prospective payment for services, based on diagnosis-related groups (DRGs). DRGs were aimed at controlling payments made to hospitals for services provided, but did not include physician services in the payment calculation. Thus physicians were still free to bill on a fee-for-service basis. In 1990, Medicare initiated resource-based relative value scales, a prospective payment mechanism for physician services that shifted the emphasis to primary care and reduced payments for certain specialty care services.

As the financing and organization of medical care became more complex in the 1970s and 1980s, hospitals and physicians began experimenting with horizontal integration by adding related, and sometimes unrelated ancillary businesses, as a means of maintaining market share and economic performance. The introduction of prospective reimbursement for both hospitals and physicians further fueled new approaches to integration. Vertical integration strategies between hospitals and physicians incorporated inpatient, outpatient, and various forms of community- and home-based care services (Conrad and Hoare 1994, 2–5).

There continues to be a growing move toward more comprehensive health "systems" reform, which includes reform of the structure of the delivery system (hospital and physicians) as well as the insurance system. Health systems reform is being enacted on a piecemeal basis in many states and communities, and the anticipation of health care reform is shaping the health care industry nationwide. Shortell, Morrison, and Friedman (1990, 303) identified two major health policy themes for the 1990s: (1) making tough choices based on value added (that is, perceived quality and improvement in health status for a given cost, or lower cost for a given level of quality and improved health status); and (2) holding individuals, organizations, and systems accountable for their choices. They outlined a public policy scenario that includes the establishment of fiscal and clinical accountability; performance-based allocation of resources; and up-front negotiations of financing and delivery.

Under health care reform initiatives, there is a move toward capitated payment mechanisms that pay on a per-person-per-month basis rather than a per-procedure or fee-for-service basis. Thus health care organizations will increasingly seek to enroll large populations for which they will negotiate capitated payments. Planning for capitation will require health organizations to determine accurately their "risk" or likely expense for health care services for the population they are proposing to serve, and to price services accurately in order to negotiate competitive rates. The incentives will be to reduce costs through preventing illness, promoting health, and emphasizing primary care services rather than providing expensive tertiary care. Health services organizations will need to understand the demographic makeup and health status characteristics of the population they are contracting to serve, and learn to manage the total health care experience more effectively.

Health care delivery in the future, then, will increasingly be: (1) primary care driven; (2) geographically decentralized with multiple convenient outlets; (3) able to take care of large groups, communities, or populations; (4) dependent on sophisticated information management with a complete knowledge of all health care expenditures; and (5) required to maintain systems that monitor utilization, cost, quality, patient access, and satisfaction. Further, health care organizations will need to assume financial risk through prospective payment and capitation for all providers who serve the contracted population, and develop adequate controls without creating barriers to access. These new directions are leading hospitals and physicians to explore a variety of new types of affiliations and integration strategies.

Implicit within the move toward greater systems integration is the notion that high quality health care services can be delivered efficiently. An opposite assumption has been made in health care delivery in the past, with quality of care raised as the justification for ever-increasing cost. Health care organizations nationwide are striving to integrate systems for monitoring and evaluating the performance of their organizations with the clinical measurement systems used by practitioners who deliver care within them. Measurement is certainly not new to the clinician, who gathers a tremendous amount of data in order to diagnose patients and treat them effectively. Health care organizations have devised elaborate and highly sophisticated financial-performance measurement systems. However, data gathered through these activities have rarely been integrated.

Integrating clinical and operational data systems is enhanced by a growing body of research that links the cost of services provided for a specific diagnosis to the outcomes achieved, while evaluating the quality of that outcome within a range of expected outcomes based on acceptable medical practice. Practice patterns including the resources used, costs incurred, and outcomes achieved can be compared across institutions, communities, and regions, and even nationally. Based on these findings, inappropriate variances in practice can be reduced. Further, it will be possible to document continuous improvement in both process and output.

Shortell, Morrison, and Friedman (ibid.) postulate that, as budgetary limitations and performance expectations are determined, systems will grant considerable autonomy to local delivery sites to organize themselves as they wish. Systems that provide greater added value will attract more patients; those that cannot will experience losses. Finally, they stipulate that all relevant parties will need to participate in negotiations that establish responsibilities to certain populations. Providers who specialize in certain populations such as the indigent may increasingly join with providers predominantly serving privately insured individuals to organize care for communities that address a wide range of people and health care needs.

There is no single approach to health systems integration. However, there are general directions: (1) innovative new affiliations that may include both public and private health partners; (2) incorporating clinical and operational data into integrated, systemwide information systems; (3) a shift in emphasis from cost of services to pricing of services; (4) a shift in focus from attending to the needs of an individual consumer to monitoring and promoting the health of an enrolled population; (5) promoting health by emphasizing wellness, prevention, and primary care; (6) decreasing the use of hospital-based or institutional services; and (7) engaging in a continuing effort to link improved health outcomes with the lowest possible service costs.

As incentives shift toward promoting and maintaining health and away from delivering expensive technologies, the hospital will assume less dominance in the health care system. Ambulatory care and home-based care are becoming an independent venue for diagnosis and treatment, both for acute and long-term care services, while the concept of community-based care is growing in importance within the health care system. Consequently, hospitals and physicians will increasingly seek out new health care partners who are able to develop and provide innovative new community-based alternatives. The emphasis on the health of the community will create a renewed interest in public health practice, including epidemiological methods of assessing and monitoring community health status.

In many respects, this shift toward public health comes none too soon. Despite the success of medical science in controlling epidemics caused by infectious disease, and the sophisticated technological advances of medical care, the United States again finds itself addressing many of the public health questions faced in the past. Infectious diseases such as AIDS and venereal disease are a plague affecting the globe. Other increases in mortality and morbidity are linked with problems such as poor nutrition, the use of tobacco, inadequate physical exercise, and homelessness or inadequate housing. Costs to the nation for these health problems, which are considered preventable, are in excess of $70 billion a year. Thus, management of health care and related costs is a much broader issue than slowing the escalation of costs associated with medical advances and high-technology health care.

Summary

Health care delivery has experienced substantial and rapid change since its early public health beginnings. The sophistication of health care interventions is surpassed only by the complexity of the health care problems and challenges to which they must be applied. Yet, the capacity of health care service delivery organizations to sustain the promises afforded by innovative new technology and techniques will ultimately need to depend on the rational allocation of scarce resources through integrative strategies within the delivery system. Those strategies will, of necessity, bring together public health, with its emphasis on sustaining the health of communities, and the technological prowess of medical care. Leaders of the future will need to use population-based thinking and strategies for resource allocation and problem solving, be able to understand both clinical and managerial processes, and be prepared to manage for change for some time to come.

References

Conrad, D. C., and G. Hoare. 1994. *Strategic Alignment: Managing Integrated Health Systems*. Ann Arbor, MI: Health Administration Press / AUPHA.

Haglund, C. L., and W. L. Dowling. 1993. "The Hospital." In *Introduction to Health Services*, Fourth Edition, edited by S. J. Williams and P. R. Torrens, 134–42. Albany, NY: Delmar.

Health Insurance Association of America. 1986. *Sourcebook of Health Insurance Data: 1984–1985*, Washington D.C.: The Association.

Shortell, S. M., E. Morrison, and B. Friedman. 1990. *Strategic Choices for America's Hospitals*. San Francisco, CA: Jossey-Bass.

Sonnefeld, S. T., D. R. Waldo, J. A. Lemieux, and D. R. McKusick. Fall 1991. "Projections of National Health Expenditures Through the Year 2000." *Health Care Financing Review* 13 (1): 1–27.

Torrens, P. R. 1993. "Historical Evolution and Overview of Health Services in the United States." In *Introduction to Health Services*, Fourth Edition, edited by S. J. Williams and P. R. Torrens, 1–13. Albany, NY: Delmar.

The Integration of Health System Organizations

by Austin Ross

Within the health care marketplace, provider organizations tend to move from one level to succeeding levels. The organizations that are most highly integrated are typically involved in stage four. The first stage of the health care marketplace, which in years past has been the typical environment in which care is purchased, offers care on a fee-for-service basis. The individual or organizational provider establishes the fees for specific services, until competition forces the supplier to offer or accept discounts from the "retail" fees. In stage one, insurance companies and other purchasers of health service (for example, employers) attempt to contain health care costs and provide services to their groups through strategies that do not attempt to change the basic methods through which care is delivered. Solo practice is still viable, and the patient has full freedom of choice of physicians and hospitals. The health care delivery system consists of independent physicians, group practices, hospitals, skilled nursing facilities, and other organizational arrangements.

In the second stage, purchasers become more sophisticated and create incentives to providers to collaborate to achieve certain purchaser objectives. A purchaser may assure a provider, for example, that if it agrees to provide services for a predetermined rate, the purchaser will direct an additional volume of patients to that provider, which will therefore achieve a marketing advantage. Exclusivity is an organizational arrangement in stage two, creating a preferred provider status. The purchaser selects a panel of providers and excludes others.

Stage three is an extension of stage two and involves more tightly defined arrangements. In the third stage, providers begin to assume financial risks for providing care. An amount is established for which a provider will care for patients on an enrollee basis (capitated care). The rate is global rather than based on fee-for-service. If the provider incurs costs greater than the capitated amount per enrollee, the provider assumes a loss for a contract term. If, on the other hand, care is provided for less than the capitated amount, the provider keeps the difference. Hospitals and physicians are encouraged to share proportionate degrees of risk. Integrated systems that are sharing risk tend either to establish an insurance mechanism of their own so that they can manage the risk themselves or to align themselves with insurance companies or other organizations to achieve the desired risk-management capacity.

In stage three, the market defines price through capitation mechanisms. Systems work to eliminate excess capacity. The disappearance of fee-for-service payment structures leaves providers with minimal capacity to shift costs. (Cost shifting is defined as transferring losses incurred under certain contracts to other payers who will to pay more generously.) The market demands a high level of exclusivity, and arrangements between providers and purchasers extend over long contract periods.

The fourth stage can be identified as the stage of accountable care. In this stage, integrated health care delivery systems define services based on population demographics. The integrated system provides to groups of the population a full range of health care services, from health education and illness prevention, through acute and chronic care. The demographics of the served population becomes the driver, and the organization's health care strategies are designed to approach the total care of the patient rather than a particular condition or episode of illness.

In stage four, the provider of care (the integrated delivery system) becomes accountable for the quality of care, service, and access. The purchaser of care has increased power to select providers, since the overall performance of the provider becomes more public. "Report cards" compare patient satisfaction and other clinical indexes. Contract decisions are based on demonstrated value, which includes quality and price. (The "four-step market stage classification" is adapted from a 1994 article on VHA's explorations of integration strategies) (Lutz 1994).

Governance, Structure, and Organizational Characteristics

As organizations advance through degrees of integration, shifts take place in their governance and management structures. In an early stage of integration, interorganizational relationships (structure, authority, and accountability) are loosely defined. As integration increases, corporate structures become more complex, often with multiple boards and intricate reporting relationships. A regrouping of functions and assignments often occurs in more integrated models. Organizational structures are flattened, functions are simplified, and control is centralized.

The physician's role also tends to change as integration increases. Physicians are involved in multiple levels of decision making in integrated systems.

In earlier stages of integration, the physician's role is typically limited to clinical intervention. In the advanced model, the physician is involved both at the clinical management level and at the broader management and governance levels, and the organizational focus also shifts from the performance of individual physicians to comparisons of health outcomes. Expanded databases and the establishment of external bench marks concentrate on the health status of the population served.

Elements of an Integrated Delivery System

There are a number of elements common to most successful integrated delivery systems. The following are particularly noteworthy.

A competent governance and management structure. The process of merging cultures and aligning interests as organizations group together is complex. The organizations that prosper are those that pay careful attention to structuring governance and management. The effect of the new organization on existing governance and management processes should be considered early in the process and is of the highest priority. Mergers and alliances that fail probably didn't pay enough attention to the merging of governance and management processes.

An involved medical staff. This is of particular importance. Physician involvement in the integrated system occurs at two levels. The first is governance and management. Organizations that do not understand the need for high-level physician involvement will typically find their paths obstructed by physician resistance. Physicians need to be full partners and leaders in the delivery of health care. The second level is clinical. Physician practice patterns can differ widely. It is the ability and competence of the medical staff leadership that will make the difference in demonstrating the value of integration.

Multiple services offered under one organizational umbrella. Integrated delivery systems work most effectively and efficiently when they control the elements in the chain of services: primary, secondary, and tertiary care; preventive services; education; and the ability to care for chronically ill patients. The integrated delivery system does not have to own all of the components, but it must have some level of control over them in order to coordinate care and provide continuity of care through a spectrum of medical activities.

An alignment of professional and system interests. Budding integrated systems often flounder because of lack of attention to the alignment of professional and system interests. A common sense of mission and a jointly held vision of where the system should be heading are critical. It is also important that the financial interests of the parties be aligned.

A focus on primary care. Primary care provides the organization with the capacity to provide broad-based services to defined population groups. Ideally, the ratio of primary care specialists to other specialists is close to one-to-one. Primary care specialists include family practitioners, general medicine internists, pediatricians, and obstetricians.

A willingness to take on capitation risks. The integrated delivery system must be willing to assume a full range of capitation risks. As noted earlier, in order to do so the system must have some basic control over the elements involved in the provision of care. Taking on risks can be an expensive learning process, but is key to a successful idea system. Incentives to manage and coordinate care are sharpened when one is at financial risk for the outcome.

Comprehensive data systems. A significant weakness in current systems is the difficulty of merging their clinical and financial data systems. Data systems tend to be segmented and poorly coordinated. Integrated delivery systems invest substantial capital in correcting this deficiency as they mature.

A long-range strategy to assume responsibility for the health status of population groups. The incorporation of population-based demographics in making decisions about how best to provide care to defined population groups is still a little-used methodology. The integrated delivery systems of the future will assess the total health of the population served as contrasted with the traditional focus on just the acute or episodic care of a single patient.

Ownership or joint venture of an insurance mechanism. The integrated delivery system needs to be fully engaged in insurance practices for it to determine risks and price services under capitation and managed care principles.

A highly coordinated and continuous strategic planning cycle. Successful integrated delivery systems recognize that planning is a continuous process rather than a static one. Multiple variables in the marketplace require that the organization's direction be constantly assessed and its planning fine-tuned.

Adequate capitalization. Capital is a significant driver. The incentive for organizations to group together is often the capital that is generated by such consolidations, mergers, or alliances. Significant capital is needed, for example, to develop the necessary sophisticated data and information systems, to acquire practices needed to develop primary care networks, and to capitalize insurance products properly.

Selected System Models

Integrated health care delivery systems may take a number of widely varying forms. The following models represent only the major categories.

Networks of Single-Specialty Groups

From 1980 to 1991, the number of physicians in single-specialty group practices nearly doubled to 76,143, or 45 percent of all physicians in group practices. (Jakleric 1994, 71). The main incentive for the specialist in a managed care market is survival, and the regional and national networking of single-specialty group practices is a significant trend. The objective of these new special care networks is to increase access to patients through the development of regional and national contracts with the purchasers of care (e.g., large employers and insurance companies).

Typically, purchasers of care from these new networks select groups that have a history of organizational stability, demonstrate activity in clinical research, and are willing to standardize critical pathways (manage care). Generally, the organization wishing to form a single-specialty group expects its members to invest capital in the venture, meet certain performance criteria, and participate actively in programs to reduce cost and ensure high quality. Arrangements typically call for an annual performance review to maintain membership.

Clinics without Walls

A clinic without walls (CWW) is a federation of individual groups and practices that agree to share certain expenses and jointly contract with purchasers to provide service at agreed-upon reimbursement schedules. Assets and practices are typically owned by the practicing physicians. Hospitals also often sponsor CWWs.

The primary objective is to provide a collective base for gaining access to patients through arrangements with insurance companies and others. A CWW provides marketing advantages in an immature managed care environment, protects the autonomy of its affiliated practices, offers a training ground for further networking and the assumption of additional risks in capitation, and represents a reasonably low-risk first step in the continuum of integration.

It is very difficult, however, for a CWW to attain sufficient practice efficiencies over a period of time. The CWW can lack marketing effectiveness, particularly when competing with a more integrated system, and may find it difficult to document quality because of the diversity of data collection systems. Further, it is often difficult for a CWW to develop practice guidelines because of variances in practice patterns among the physicians involved.

While a few years ago the CWW was considered a prominent model for integrated delivery of health care, the future of CWWs today seems quite limited in light of the advantages of more highly integrated systems.

Management Service Organizations

The management service organization (MSO) represents a higher level of integration. It provides a highly visible coordinated system that is centrally accountable for performance and therefore allegedly more attractive to purchasers of care. MSOs may be sponsored by hospitals, jointly ventured between physicians and hospitals, or operated as freestanding entities. Their key feature is a central management. Assets are generally, but not always, owned by the organization.

While still affording some autonomy to the physician, MSOs attain perceived additional practice efficiencies through centralization. The organizational structure enhances the marketing of services (as a more cohesive delivery system), and provides access to capital.

On the down side, MSOs may encounter legal and inurement issues relating to aspects of ownership by physicians. MSOs find it difficult to define a central culture or mission for the organization. They can be dominated by an inpatient focus, which may be detrimental in terms of developing contractual arrangements, and MSOs may be less efficient than more mature models for delivering care.

MSOs may well, however, provide core elements for larger regional systems. Their future is relatively secure in the evolution of these systems. The management service organization is very similar in structure and function to the physician hospital organization.

Medical Foundation Model

The medical foundation model usually consists of a 501(c)(3) nonprofit organization with employed physicians. The operation is centrally controlled and managed, and highly integrated, and the foundation typically owns the assets. Its objectives, as with the other models, are to achieve operating efficiencies and provide the full spectrum of health care. The foundation model is in a strong position to do so. Its primary advantages include the economy-of-scale efficiencies associated with a highly integrated organization; its access to capital, which enables the system to maintain technology and expand; its assumption of the financial risk, which relieves the physician of investment requirements; and the fact that it is well positioned for capitation arrangements with third party payers.

The disadvantages of a foundation model include the concern that there is less physician autonomy; the restrictions, both clinical and administrative, that the organization will tend to impose on its physician complement; and a cumbersome decision-making process, attributable to community control of the board or parent organization as required of not-for-profit organizations eligible for tax exemption. Additionally, there may be an obligation to the community, such that some of the proceeds may need to flow back into the community.

As for the future, the medical foundation model may represent the best option for long-term survival. These organizations will mature into tightly integrated structures providing the full range of health care services under one umbrella.

Internal Assessment

An organization, such as a group practice, that wants to move toward higher levels of integration needs to perform several internal and external assessments, beginning with a complete internal profile of the organization, its growth, the age of its medical staff, the marketplace, the competition, and so forth. Essential next are a clear understanding of how the aggregate health care system in the region is currently structured and operating and an understanding of the health care needs of the community. The organization should ensure it has the capacity to tabulate accurately the cost and quality of the services it provides in a fashion that allows and encourages comparisons with other organizations. Knowing the market share of the various organizations in the region that provide services under capitated arrangements is a must. The organization must know its own history of medical politics, in order to anticipate possible barriers to and incentives for linking with others. The organization should assess its relationships with local hospitals, with an eye toward which hospitals might make good partners. Finally, it should consider its relationships with private and public agencies, as cooperation between the private and public sectors can often open new avenues of positive joint venturing.

In short, the organization preparing for integration needs to conduct a thorough inventory to determine eligible partners, goals and obstacles, appropriate partners, and the appropriate mix of physicians and other providers.

Getting Ready to Engage in Processes of Integration

There are a number of steps an organization can take to prepare itself for integration. These include

- Simplifying and flattening the management structure.
- Empowering lower levels of the organization to make decisions to free up time for the senior executives to evaluate the potential integration arrangement.
- Solving system problems through processes of simplification (continuous quality improvement).
- Ensuring that physicians are totally involved and not left by the sidelines.
- Rethinking reporting practices to strengthen operations and reserve time for strategic issues.
- Upgrading management competency at every level.
- Defining corporate culture to help prepare for selecting appropriate partners. (The majority of failures in mergers, affiliations, or alliances can be tracked back to the lack of corporate cultural compatibility.)
- Refining mission and vision statements to ensure that the organization has clear direction.
- Ensuring that strategic planning is continual rather than static.

Summary

There are a growing number of integrated health care delivery systems. These systems are developing in response to market forces in anticipation of legislative changes at the federal level. Even without sweeping legislative changes, these systems will continue to expand in the several years ahead. Competition will be fierce, and health care delivery organizations will be confronted with multiple choices in the selection of partners. Rural America will also be affected by these changes, although initially at a slower pace.

References

Jakleric, M. C. 1994. "Staying Single: Can Single Specialty Group Practices Survive in Managed Care Markets?" *Modern Health Care* 24 (40): 71–80.

Lutz, S. 1994. "VHA. Set to Take Executives to the School of Successful Strategies for Integration." *Modern Health Care* 24 (31): 84–8.

Integrating Public Health and Medicine
Creating a Community Health Focus

by Katharine Sacks Sanders and Mary Richardson

The debate on health care reform in the United States has focused a great deal of attention on the importance of integrating public health and medicine, two fields that have operated separately for nearly a century (Starr 1982). Health care policy debates have sparked considerable change and realignment in health care financing and delivery nationwide, even in the absence of reform legislation. Such changes are producing a shift away from fee-for-service payment methodologies, which offer financial incentives to provide more rather than fewer services, to capitated financing mechanisms, which reward the delivery of fewer rather than more services. Under capitation, providers contract to provide services to a community of people, receiving payment on a per-person basis depending on the number of persons enrolled by the provider. Payment remains the same regardless of the number of services provided.

As financing mechanisms shift from fee-for-service to capitation payment models, there is a growing emphasis on improving health in an effort to reduce service utilization. Managing the health of people, rather than serving them once they become ill or injured, is a significant shift in focus for many health care delivery organizations. The incentives within the system are realigned toward reduced use of intensive, expensive services and promoting strategies for maintaining or improving personal health. Since individual health is affected by health, social, and economic conditions in the larger community, the shift in incentives requires a better understanding of the health status of the community as a whole. Health status improvements, measured by regular health assessments, provide documentation and demonstrate public accountability (Quality Letter for Healthcare Leaders 1994).

The concept of healthy communities, with its emphasis on planning and managing the health of a target population, is capturing the attention of health care delivery organizations across the country. Managing community health will require different types of provider organizations working together using various integrating mechanisms.

Population-based planning and health promotion have traditionally been public health rather than medical care activities. Meeting the new challenges facing health care delivery organizations will require physicians, hospitals, health departments, community health agencies, and other components of the delivery system, which have functioned in parallel but quite separate ways until now, to integrate.

History of Public Health

The roots of the United States health care system are within public health practice. The health of Americans was in early times compromised by epidemics of acute, infectious, and highly lethal disease. Crowded living conditions in the cities, a result of industrialization and rapid growth, increased the spread of illness and death. During the 1800s, public health efforts concentrated on improving sanitation. Ill people were routinely quarantined to control the spread of disease. Development of the sciences of bacteriology and pathology in the late 1800s, along with more effective systems for water purification, disposal of sewage, and monitoring and safeguarding food, and the improving quality of urban housing, combined to bring epidemics of acute infectious disease under control by the turn of the nineteenth century.

After 1900, health problems such as pneumonia and tuberculosis took the place of massive epidemics as the target of medical attention. These problems spurred the development of immunization programs and efforts to prevent the transmission of infectious diseases such as tuberculosis and venereal diseases including syphilis. By 1925, most of the causes and methods of transmission of leading communicable diseases had been identified. With the advent of antibiotics in the 1940s, chronic diseases replaced acute infectious diseases as the primary cause of death. Healthier living conditions and a decline in infectious disease allowed people to live longer. Conditions such as heart disease, cancer, and stroke become more prevalent in the population, accounting for nearly two-thirds of all deaths by 1990.

The increasing sophistication of bacteriologic and pathologic science also created a growing appreciation of the importance of appropriate laboratory facilities to determine the prevalence of communicable disease agents among the population or in the environment. Public health, generally thought to fall within the jurisdiction of the states, became an important governmental function across the country. By 1909, all states had organized some type of health department and had established jurisdiction over the management of public health.

Health departments were also organized at the city or county level, often under voluntary boards. They were staffed by public health professionals and led by public health physicians. The relationship between local health departments and the state varied, depending on state legislation and organizational structure. This variation from state to state continues today. Then, as now, major areas of public health activity generally included control of communicable disease, operation of public health laboratories, assurance of the safety of food and water supplies, collection and management of vital statistics, and provision of certain services such as health education, immunizations, and home visits.

Public Health and Personal Health Services

As cities grew and public health problems related to immigration and population growth increased, public services struggled to keep up with sanitation, housing, and water needs. Public health departments became providers of last resort for people without resources to pay for medical care. Following funding patterns, personal health services were targeted to specific services such as maternal and child health, venereal disease, and tuberculosis detection.

Health departments today generally provide both clinical and environmental services. Clinical services typically include prenatal care, infant and well-child care, child growth and development programs, immunization, and infectious and chronic disease surveillance. Some may also provide occupational health programs for local government employees. Environmental services generally include sewage-disposal systems, food and restaurant inspections, animal control, and mosquito control. There is a growing emphasis in many health departments on waste disposal and attention to ground, water, and air pollution.

Public Health Careers and Professions

Professional preparation for public health careers developed in the late 1800s. The leaders of the day saw the growing field of medical science as the basis for training in the practice of the science and arts of public health (Acheson 1990). The Massachusetts Institute of Technology (MIT) and Harvard University, moved by the efforts of biologist William Sedgewick, jointly created the degree of Doctor of Public Health. Public health students shared preclinical instruction with those seeking the Doctor of Medicine degree, and then moved into a course of study that included preventive medicine, vital statistics, sanitary science and preventive sanitation, public health laboratory methods, epidemiology, preventive hygiene (e.g., mental, social, personal, and dental hygiene), and public health education and administration. Medical students, on the other hand, went to the hospital wards to complete their education.

The MIT-Harvard Doctorate in Public Health flourished until 1922, and other universities created similar programs. However, over time the medical component was separated from public health training, and general medicine became the dominant force in the U.S. health care system. Significantly greater financial rewards, the prestige of medical training, and the absence of public health philosophy in medical training are cited as factors that contributed to medical dominance over public health (ibid.). As personal health care services grew in importance for health departments, practitioners of general medicine began to protect against the potential encroachment of public health services into their own practices. Public health services continued to focus primarily on communitywide issues such as the management of communicable disease and the provision of services to the indigent or other individuals who could not afford to pay for care.

Public Health Funding

Significant federal funding of public health at the state level began with the passage of the Social Security Act of 1935, which created a grant-in-aid program to provide support for state and local health departments. These funds included grants specific to the provision of maternal and child health services (Title V) and general funds for the development of state and local health initiatives (Title VI). States were required to match federal dollars. As public health departments increased in number, and services proliferated, a special committee of the American Public Health Association (APHA), chaired by Dr. Haven Emerson, developed a set of standards for assessing the existence of minimally adequate public health services. These standards addressed staffing, types of services to be offered, the organization of services, and other similar issues (Roemer 1993).

Over time, health departments have grown in size and scope. Due to government-financed insurance through Medicare and Medicaid and the proliferation of health care technology, general medicine has also expanded. The two systems, however, have grown primarily in a parallel, somewhat disconnected fashion. Both systems continue to offer personal care services, with the public health system generally serving people who have limited financial resources, and the general medical system serving the insured population.

Over the last decade, more and more people have found themselves without health insurance or other financial resources to pay for care. In an attempt to fill the gap, public health agencies have offered increasing numbers of personal care services. The public health system thus tends to provide care to people who are more vulnerable, whose health status is more fragile, and whose social and economic circumstances make them more challenging to serve. The targeted nature of public health funding, however, often restricts the types of services available to these groups. Federally funded rural, community, and migrant health care centers offer more comprehensive services, but their availability is limited, and most local public health agencies offer little primary care for noninfectious diseases or chronic conditions.

Reform of the Public Health System

The shift for public health will be substantial in a reformed system. A 1988 Institute of Medicine (IOM) study of the public health system concluded that the public health system is in disarray (Committee for the Study 1988). The study found tremendous differences among state and local public health agencies in the functions they perform and in the services they provide. One of the most significant conclusions was that the focus on personal health services for people without access to other medical care has diverted public health resources and attention away from critical services such as communicable disease prevention and surveillance, leaving many communities vulnerable once again to infectious diseases such as measles and tuberculosis. In addition, a lack of resources for health education and health promotion, widely accepted as public health activities, has contributed to the spread of HIV/AIDS. The IOM defined the mission of public health as "fulfilling society's interest in assuring conditions in which people can be healthy," and recommended that public health agencies rededicate themselves to the core functions of community health assessment and policy development, assuring only that essential personal medical services be provided.

In 1993, the APHA adopted a vision of a reformed system that incorporates the major IOM recommendations. As shown in Figure 1 below, much of the current overlap of the public and personal health systems in the areas of clinical preventive and personal medical services would be eliminated in the reformed health system, and public health would focus primarily on community prevention programs. Achieving this vision will require major changes in the allocation of public health resources and funding systems. States such as Washington, Montana, and Georgia are working to adapt and implement this vision locally.

Figure 1

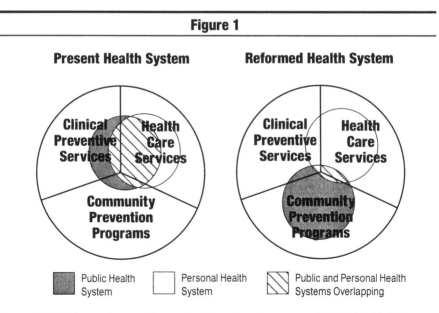

Present Health System

Reformed Health System

Clinical Preventive Services

Health Care Services

Community Prevention Programs

Clinical Preventive Services

Health Care Services

Community Prevention Programs

Public Health System   Personal Health System   Public and Personal Health Systems Overlapping

From: APHA Subcommittee on Community Prevention Programs and Public Health Vision, "APHA's Vision: Public Health and a Reformed Health Care System," *The Nation's Health*, July 1993, pp. 9–11.

Moving toward Integration

Much of the debate around health care reform from the consumer perspective has centered on the issue of choice of a provider. Nearly 40 million Americans have had that choice reduced or eliminated because they are uninsured. The public health system has, in many instances, been their only choice unless they entered the general medical system through a hospital emergency room. However, financial access is only one of the barriers for this population. Population groups with limited access to the general medical care system in the United States today include:

1. Low-income groups and individuals who have little education
2. Members of certain racial, cultural, and ethnic groups and those who speak languages other than English
3. Residents of inner-city, rural, and extremely geographically isolated (frontier) communities
4. Individuals and families who lack a stable residence, such as migrant workers and the homeless
5. Adolescents
6. Individuals with chronic health conditions such as HIV / AIDS, mental illness, disability-related conditions, and chemical dependency

If access is changed and the uninsured are brought into the personal care system in the private sector, people who fall into the categories listed above and who are currently uninsured will not only be "added," but under the various health care reform designs being implemented by the states, they will be "shifted away" from the public health system. The challenge will be to integrate these populations effectively into the evolving personal care system. With the growing emphasis on population-based approaches to health care delivery, and the need for better strategies to serve vulnerable populations, hospital-physician-community alliances are already beginning to form. It is the "community" portion of this integration that most often involves the public sector of health care.

The IOM study, the American Public Health Association, the Council on Scientific Affairs of the American Medical Association, the American Hospital Association, the Healthcare Forum, and numerous other groups and individuals have urged increased collaboration among private and public health care providers to improve community health status, reduce duplication of services, and contain costs.

The Council on Scientific Affairs report on public health describes some of the barriers that may exist between public health and private physicians (Council on Scientific Affairs 1990). It is likely that many persons in each group do not understand the essential significance of the other group to the community's well-being. Physicians in public health may be viewed as being unable to perform the usual techniques and procedures of physicians in clinical practice. Yet health department officials must be capable of carrying out other kinds of procedures, such as preparing a multimillion-dollar budget or investigating a food-borne epidemic. Physicians in public health, who are working for the good of the community at large, may view private practitioners more as businesspersons than as physicians.

The report suggests that, to ameliorate the situation, physicians in public health and those in private practice should consider consulting with one another on such topics as immunizations and communicable diseases. Another suggestion is that clinicians consider studying in depth one or more of the "diverse subjects of public health" or volunteering to assist a public health agency.

Public health agencies depend directly on local political processes for a significant portion of their funding. Many receive 40 percent or more of their funds from local city or county governments, or both. Thus, their effectiveness in addressing perceived community health issues and publicizing improvements directly affects their budgets. Yet often they are expected to address multifaceted community issues such as teen pregnancy and violence, problems that public health professionals cannot resolve by themselves. Even "cooperation" with other health care providers alone will not resolve these issues. However, hospitals and health systems often have ties with influential community members who can help bring in the resources of business and service group leaders; public health leaders tend to have relationships with schools, social service providers, and at-risk populations that private health care providers may not have. Together, the two groups often have the expertise and influence to mobilize the larger efforts required to make significant progress on complex community issues.

Cooperative, integrative efforts among personal health care providers and public health agencies range from short-term cosponsorship of health promotion activities such as public service announcements about healthy lifestyles (Healthy Cities), to providing shared comprehensive health services for underserved groups (Lumsdon 1993), to assumption of major public health responsibilities by private providers in some rural communities, to ongoing collaboration for community health status assessment, intervention, and evaluation as part of broad community coalitions.

The shape and pace of collaborative efforts are determined by a variety of factors, including local and regional public health and personal health care resources (professional, technical, information systems, financial); the relationship of public health to Medicaid administration in the state bureaucracy; and the level of competition between the public and private sectors. The history of community collaboration and the personalities of key health care leaders also contribute.

Collaborative efforts may be easier to manage in most rural areas than in urban communities. Rural areas often have traditions of cooperation based on a recognition that scarce resources will go further in meeting community needs if organizations and individuals work together. For example, a small rural hospital in Iowa was able to enhance its health promotion efforts by absorbing the community health section of the county health department into its operations. The public health nurse manager added the functions of hospital nurse manager when she joined the staff (Kernaghan 1992).

Evolving systems in rural areas of Idaho (Magic Valley) and Washington State (Southwest Washington Medical Center and Southwest Washington Health District) are bringing public health administrators onto hospital and health system boards and strategic planning committees. Hospital and system administrators, in turn, are serving on public health advisory boards. In this way, local public health agencies and medical providers are bringing the influence and perspective of their counterparts into their own policymaking apparatus.

Building on a number of collaborative and streamlining efforts among five rural hospitals in Washington State, two public hospital districts in Lincoln County developed a public health coalition to provide public health personal care services for the county. The county commissioners requested that the hospitals, which are respected major employers in the area, take on this function. Environmental health services remain with the county. Public health staff are now employees of the new public health coalition, and public health services are being supplemented by nursing services once devoted exclusively to acute hospital care. The hospital districts continue to be involved in larger regional efforts to assess and improve community health status.

Large hospitals and health systems such as Mount Sinai Hospital Medical Center in Chicago and the Morton Plant System in Clearwater, Florida have used community partnerships to assess needs and target resources to improve health. Along with the Salvation Army and the Pinellas County Health Department, the Morton Plant system is developing a comprehensive health care program for indigent mothers and their children (Lumsdon 1993). Organizers say it took six months for the Morton Plant system and the health department representatives to understand how one another operated and to develop guidelines for the program.

Summary

With or without legislated health care reform, the growing emphasis on the health of the community will form the basis for innovative approaches to integration of medical care and public health services. Shifts in financing mechanisms and the pressure to contain costs provide substantial incentives for hospitals and personal health care providers to focus on community health improvement. A community effort to reduce teenage drinking and driving, for example, can bring down the costs of trauma care for motor vehicle injuries. Growing public concern about accountability will also promote integration. Health care delivery organizations are being asked, more and more, to account to the American public for the resources they use and the quality of the health outcomes they produce. This is especially important for nonprofit hospitals and health care systems that must demonstrate that they are "earning" their tax-exempt status by making worthwhile contributions to the community. The greatest incentive, however, may be the growing recognition that medical and technological interventions alone cannot adequately promote health within a population. It is the tools of public health — community health assessment and policy development — combined with medicine and technology, that will lead to creative new partnerships and, ultimately, improved health outcomes.

References

APHA Subcommittee on Community Prevention Programs and Public Health Vision. 1993. "APHA's Vision: Public Health and a Reformed Health Care System." *The Nation's Health* Vol. XXIII, No. VI: 9–11.

Acheson, R. M. 1990. "The Medicalization of Public Health; the United Kingdom and the United States Contrasted." *Journal of Public Health Medicine* 12 (1): 31–38.

Committee for the Study of the Future of Public Health, Division of Health Care Services, Institute of Medicine. 1988. *The Future of Public Health*. Washington, D.C.: The Institute.

Council on Scientific Affairs. 1990. "The IOM Report and Public Health." *Journal of the American Medical Association* 264 (4): 503–6.

Kernaghan, S. G. 1992. *Healthy People 2000 in Rural America: Hospitals and Communities Rally*. Chicago: American Hospital Association.

Lumsdon, K. 1993. "Patience and Partnership: Health Systems Cultivate Two Ingredients to Create Healthier Communities." *Hospitals and Health Care Networks* 67 (24): 26–31.

Roemer, M. I. 1993. "Joseph W. Mountin, Architect of Modern Public Health." *Public Health Reports* 108 (6): 727–35.

Starr, P. 1982. *The Social Transformation of American Medicine*. New York: Harper Collins.

Veatch, R. 1994. *The Quality Letter for Healthcare Leaders*. Bader & Associates, Inc. 6(5).

PART III

The Organization

System Organization
and Integration

The Community Clinical Oncology Program
The Case of Oxford Medical Center

by Arnold D. Kaluzny, W. Paul Kory, and Dan Garson-Angert

Over the past 30 years in the United States, there has been a dramatic change in the provision of cancer care in local communities. The recognition that 80 percent of all cancer is treated in local communities (Greenwald, Cullen, and McKenna 1987) resulted in the implementation of a program designed to ensure that state-of-the-art technology for cancer treatment and control was available to community physicians. The Community Clinical Oncology Program (CCOP) is designed to bring the benefits of treatment and cancer prevention and control research to patients in local communities by enabling community physicians to enroll patients in clinical trials that previously were available only through major centers for cancer treatment and research.

Figure 1 presents the CCOP network, consisting of three major components (Kaluzny, Morrissey, and McKinney 1990): the individual CCOPs, their designated research bases, and the Division of Cancer Prevention and Control of the National Cancer Institute (NCI). CCOPs are the organizational units that conduct research on cancer treatment and control at the community level. They typically consist of one or more community hospitals and a group of oncologists and other medical specialists who admit cancer patients to these hospitals. Although the hospitals may provide some financial and staff support, most of the administrative, data management, and travel costs associated with entering patients in cancer research studies are paid through cooperative agreements with the National Cancer Institute. CCOP physicians register patients and assign them to clinical trials through research bases with which the CCOP is

Based on material obtained from the NCI-funded evaluation of the Community Clinical Oncology Program (Kaluzny, Warnecke, and Gillings 1992).

Figure 1. Components of the Community Clinical Oncology Program

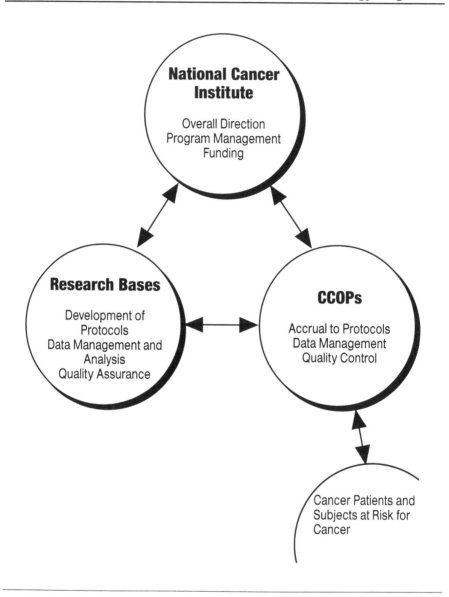

affiliated. For each patient enrolled in a research base protocol, the CCOP receives a certain amount of accrual credit. Because a typical assignment is one accrual credit per enrolled patient, CCOPs must enroll about 50 patients per year in cancer treatment protocols to meet the NCI minimum requirement of 50 accrual credits.

Each CCOP is headed by a clinician-principal investigator or coinvestigators who are responsible for the management of the CCOP activities. One or more data managers — usually nurses specializing in oncology — manage the flow of patient data between CCOP physicians and research bases and assist the physicians in identifying protocol-eligible patients. One of the incentives built into the CCOP cooperative agreements is support for physicians, data managers, and hospital support staff to attend research base scientific meetings. These meetings provide opportunities for physicians and staff to learn about new research, participate in protocol design, and develop skills in clinical trials management.

Research bases design the protocols for the treatment clinical trials and cancer control research studies in which CCOPs and other research institutions participate. In this leadership role, they also collect, verify, and analyze study data; provide training in the management of clinical trials and cancer control research; and monitor the patient enrollments and data quality of CCOPs and other research base members. Research bases may be clinical cooperative groups, core grant cancer centers, or state health departments funded by the National Cancer Institute. Each CCOP may affiliate with up to five eligible research bases, only one of which may be a national, multispecialty cooperative group.

The Division of Cancer Prevention and Control is a constituent part of the National Cancer Institute, one of the National Institutes of Health. Through its Community Oncology and Rehabilitation Branch, the Division of Cancer Prevention and Control establishes directions for the CCOP, provides funding to CCOPs and research bases, and monitors program progress. The Division of Cancer Prevention and Control staff also work with the National Cancer Institute's Division of Cancer Treatment to review and approve proposed cancer research protocols and to monitor the scientific value, quality, and provisions for patient safety of these studies.

Goals of the CCOP at Oxford

The physicians and staff at the CCOP at Oxford Medical Center agree that the major goals of the CCOP are to provide state-of-the-art care to patients with cancer living in Oxford's service area and to participate in clinical research. Other goals included changing the standard of practice among physicians at Oxford, providing cancer control activities and participating in cancer control research, and improving minorities' access to cancer care. Both the principal investigator, Dr. Smith, and the coprincipal investigator, Dr. Jones, define cancer prevention and control research as a major aim of the CCOP but also express considerable dissatisfaction with the projects presently available. (See the appendix for a listing of people associated with the CCOP.)

The Oxford CCOP has used a variety of methods to achieve its primary goal of accruing patients in treatment protocols. An important strategy has been the constant effort of Dr. Smith and other CCOP staff members to educate the medical community at Oxford, as well as at the affiliated hospitals throughout the state and region. Dr. Smith has made multiple trips to the hospitals affiliated with Oxford to present at meetings, see patients in the clinics, and speak with physicians at these other hospitals. Other participating physicians such as Drs. Selling, Peters, and Williams have also presented formally and informally at the affiliated hospitals.

At Oxford, Dr. Smith and other participating physicians regularly speak to physicians formally (e.g., at tumor board and other conferences) and informally concerning the CCOP and the availability of protocols. Nurse oncologists have been brought into the CCOP to teach house staff including a large group of family practice residents and other health care personnel about cancer treatment and control protocols. The CCOP office has started to provide all interested physicians, including primary care physicians and surgeons, with notebooks containing brief fact sheets on all the protocols available; this information is regularly updated. The CCOP data managers are now obtaining all cancer diagnoses from pathology; from that information, they are sending out letters to the physician caring for the patient describing the available protocols. Drs. Smith and Jones have attempted to generate interest among the Oxford surgeons by sending representatives to major research base meetings. The physicians participating in the CCOP receive biweekly or monthly feedback concerning their own and the other active members' accrual of patients in the context of the regular minutes passed out at the meetings. More general information concerning the availability of cancer protocols is given to the general and medical communities through hospital newsletters and a magazine.

The Oxford administrative staff — including Alice Johnson, the president; James Rice, the senior vice president for finance; and Dr. Leslie Wilson, a senior physician administrator recently named to head the cancer program at Oxford — support the CCOP in part because cancer services represent a marketable program for the hospital. The CCOP functions to legitimize the cancer-related activities at Oxford, thereby giving Oxford a competitive edge over other hospitals in the state. Other functions of the CCOP effort by Oxford have been the facilitation of referrals to treatment and cancer control protocols, institutionalization of the program at Oxford, favorable changes in physician practice patterns, and the involvement of primary care physicians in Oxford's cancer control research.

The goals of the cancer treatment protocols that exist at Oxford are outcomes of, and are reinforced by, the medical center's history of participation in protocols sponsored by four research bases, dating to the middle 1970s. A tumor registry has existed at Oxford since 1968. Dr. Williams has worked successfully to develop a statewide hospice program for children. Moreover, Oxford is attempting to develop specific guidelines for medical care generally, and will target cancer treatment for standards in the near future. Drs. Smith and Jones are part of the four-member Spearhead Group, which oversees the development of cancer guidelines. Despite the large amount of activity by CCOP members and staff, which may have had a desirable effect on the practice patterns of many community physicians, these educational activities have not been systematized or well integrated. For example, the lack of universal control protocols, and uncertainty about what constitutes cancer prevention and control, has limited the effect of educational efforts on cancer control patient accrual, and on the greater involvement of primary care physicians in cancer control research.

Program Structure

The Oxford CCOP program consists of Oxford and eight affiliated hospitals scattered throughout the state and region, most of which are too small to provide tertiary care. Together they include more than 1,000 general medical beds. Little interaction exists between the eight hospitals and Oxford; however, a few physicians at these institutions (some of whom practice primarily at Oxford) will send their patients to Oxford if an appropriate protocol is available there for their patients.

The CCOP is one of three efforts funded by grants within the cancer research department at Oxford, and the cancer research department is one part of the Cancer Research Program directed by Leslie Wilson, M.D. Oxford provides approximately $100,000 yearly in supplemental support of the Cancer Research Program.

A cancer control commission has been recently established to define the policies and provide the planning for the cancer research department. Dr. Wilson, the Cancer Research Program director, is a strong advocate for the development of clinical guidelines for all departments and physicians at Oxford. The cancer control commission, with her strong urging, has decided to pursue the development of these guidelines for the care of cancer patients by cancer site. Whether the management information system is capable of tracking the adherence of physicians to cancer clinical guidelines is not yet clear, nor is the effect on patient outcomes such adherence might have.

Recurring complaints by the physicians participating in the CCOP are that Dr. Smith fails to delegate responsibility, and that more formal organization is needed. The initial, unsuccessful CCOP grant was written by Max Steiner, the Cancer Research Program business manager, whose duties also included grant writing, while the CCOP II proposal written by Dr. Smith was approved and presently funds the CCOP. Mr. Steiner remains a dominant figure in the CCOP, controls the finances, and reviews any major expenses.

The CCOP data managers and other staff meet weekly with Dr. Smith. The data managers and other CCOP staff look to Dr. Smith for direction, and their loyalty to him is apparent. The major CCOP business is dealt with at the meeting, which also involves from 15 to 20 physicians in the CCOP. Several of the CCOP physicians, such as Dr. Jones, express a desire to exclude the CCOP staff from the meetings, but Dr. Smith strongly resists these efforts. No other CCOP committees exist. Many physicians, such as Drs. Jones and Williams, feel that

Dr. Smith makes many decisions himself prior to or between these regular meetings. There is also little formal coordination of CCOP and other activities, such as CCOP cancer control research efforts and Oxford cancer control activities. The coordination and communication that exist derive primarily from the multiple hats that many physicians and other staff wear at Oxford.

The apparent lack of formal organizational structure within the CCOP and the general dissatisfaction with the level of authority delegated to other CCOP physicians has probably undercut accrual to treatment and cancer control protocols, institutionalization, change in physician practice patterns, and the involvement of primary care physicians in cancer control research. However, Dr. Smith, who has asked Drs. Selling and Peters to head a quality control committee, and other members of the administration, such as Dr. Wilson and Dr. Doris, the chief of medicine, who have acted as mediators in the past, seem aware of these problems and are moving to address them. Dr. Smith states that he has maintained control in order to assure the quality of the program; he says past efforts to delegate duties were met with disinterest or were not carried out properly by the CCOP physicians given additional duties. Now, the rank-and-file CCOP physicians actively seek more formal organizational structure and processes for the CCOP, and several seek a more active and authoritative role in the CCOP.

Program Environment

Oxford Medical Center is in Chester County, Pennsylvania, a community of 400,000 people. The West Chester Hospital, a part of Oxford, is in one of the two largest cities in the tricounty area, a city with a minority population greater than 50 percent. The West Chester Hospital provides a large proportion of the indigent care in the tricounty area. Nearly all the hospitals in the tricounty area are affiliates of the Oxford CCOP. The catchment area includes Dover County in Delaware, Cecil County in Maryland, and Chester County in Pennsylvania; in total, approximately 2,000 hospital beds are available to one million people.

Locally, some competition with the Oxford cancer program is coming from Dover and Wilmington Hospitals; however, the main competition remains the large academic medical centers in two major metropolitan areas. A few health organizations, such as outpatient surgery operations or "doc-in-a-box" outlets, have sprung up locally in an effort to capture well-insured or paying patients from other providers.

Consumer groups, such as health maintenance organizations and business, seem to have little effect on Oxford's environment at the present time. Still, Dr. Ellens, a family physician, states that 30 percent to 40 percent of his group's patients belong to health maintenance organizations.

The regulatory environment in Pennsylvania seems stable; insurers and state government regulators are watching the many managed care initiatives that are being undertaken in other parts of the country before deciding whether to regulate or restrict them in Pennsylvania. The effort by Oxford to develop clinical guidelines is a proactive response to trends the top administrators and physicians see nationwide; that is, large hospitals will be required to implement and evaluate clinical guidelines and their clinical staff's compliance and effectiveness. Dr. Wilson thinks that moving forward with this process now, in an unhurried fashion, will allow much more efficient and effective implementation than waiting until such guidelines are mandated by insurers or government agencies.

Clinical Trials Management Procedures

At present, the Cancer Research Program, which includes the CCOP staff, has eight people supervised by Susan Harris, a registered nurse who was formerly associated with the Allegheny CCOP. Of these, seven are data managers and one is a secretary. All the data managers are registered nurses except Peter Simmons, who is a medical technologist. One part-time data manager position is unfilled. No formal educational effort exists for the data managers or other staff. Although Ms. Harris supervises all of these personnel, two of them are working solely on non-CCOP projects, and one works 60 percent of her time on CCOP. Despite their position in the hospital administrative structure, the Cancer Research Program staff members see themselves as working with Dr. Smith to carry on the various research projects.

The Cancer Research Program staff makes every effort to facilitate the enrollment and treatment of patients on National Cancer Institute protocols. In the last year, the CCOP data managers have begun to use microcomputers to maintain their patient files. The aggressive and enthusiastic tenor of the data managers is reflected in Peter Simmons' comment that their motto is, "Once randomized, always analyzed." The Cancer Research Program staff circulates protocols to the CCOP physicians for comments and review prior to the meetings; then they collect and collate the comments of the physicians and other staff. At the meetings, the physician or physicians most interested in the protocol guide it through the institutional review board, and the Cancer Research Program staff help with the submission. Dr. Smith has been the dominant force moving protocols through this process. If the institutional review board requests revisions or clarifications of a protocol, the Cancer Research Program staff assists the physicians in gathering the desired information.

When the Cancer Research Program adopts a protocol, the staff helps: (1) disseminate it to all interested parties, update it when appropriate, and answer any questions concerning it; (2) identify patients who may be eligible; (3) inform patients about it, when requested by a physician; (4) obtain necessary tests or other information concerning the protocol or specific patients for physicians' office staff or floor personnel; and (5) recognize and resolve problems due to treatment of a patient on a protocol, from reporting complications to helping obtain funding.

Ms. Harris estimates that the staff are following 350 patients in the Cancer Research Program; she thinks larger patient numbers or different duties, such as those for cancer control research, will require more personnel. (She is also unsure if the microcomputers that they now use for the clinical trial data will be sufficient for the collection of cancer control data.) Some CCOP physicians call on the Cancer Research Program staff to perform few of the latter functions, such as Dr. Ruth, a radiation therapist, while others have the data managers handle the patients and their data management completely. Most physicians deal with their patients themselves but allow the data managers to perform most of the data collection functions. Still, the relationship of the office staffs of most of the CCOP physicians and the Cancer Research Program personnel seems good. Contact between CCOP physicians and data managers is at least weekly, and in some cases daily.

Despite their success in placing high numbers of patients on protocols, Drs. Smith and Jones are not sure how large a percentage of eligible patients are placed on protocols. Dr. Williams asserts that nearly 100 percent of the children with cancer are placed on a protocol because he or Dr. Jones sees them all. Drs. Smith and Jones think that the surgeons still fail to refer many of their eligible patients for therapy. Although financial considerations have not prevented any patients from being put on a protocol as yet, Drs. Smith and Jones express concern about this in the future. Further, none of the physicians has serious problems with placing health maintenance organization patients on protocols.

The efficient, effective, and committed Cancer Research Program staff is a crucial element in the success of the CCOP program at Oxford. Although their duties have not been written formally, the management procedures that are being carried out greatly facilitate accrual to treatment and cancer control research protocols, institutionalization, change in physician practice patterns, and the involvement of primary care physicians in cancer control research. Still, all of the data managers complain that they do not receive sufficient feedback on individual patients and study outcomes.

Physician Relationships

The physicians involved in the Oxford CCOP are notable for their academic credentials and their prior associations with various clinical cooperative groups. Dr. Williams, for example, has maintained the formal association with one group, and Dr. Lawson is working closely with another cooperative group. Joshua Miles, M.D., who was an important force in cancer control research at the National Cancer Institute, has close ties to Oxford, supporting the development of the Oxford CCOP. Thus, a very strong foundation for the CCOP existed at Oxford before the program began.

Nearly all of the 12 hematology/oncology physicians in rural southeast Pennsylvania practice primarily at Oxford and have participated in protocols at Oxford. These physicians include three groups: (1) Drs. Jane's and Jones's group of five physicians, from whom Dr. Smith and his two partners split; (2) Dr. Smith's group; and (3) Drs. Peters and Selling. Dr. Bruce Williams, a pediatric hematologist/oncologist, and Dr. Lear, a low-accruing oncologist, practice alone.

Competition and a degree of ill feeling exist among some of the CCOP physicians. Drs. Peters and Selling are relatively new to the area and are still building their practice. Dr. Ruth, a radiation therapist, states that her group is the only one in rural southeastern Pennsylvania offering comprehensive radiation therapy services. Although she agrees with the major aims of the CCOP and has few conflicts with the other physicians, she is ambivalent because her group actually loses money from their involvement with protocols. She states that participation is particularly time-consuming for the radiation therapy physicians and their staff, due to the review requirements.

No formal penalties exist for failure to accrue patients or to meet quality control standards. Fortunately, no one has had poor quality control; low accruers are given public feedback and are approached informally. Physician participation is rewarded by sending high accruers to research base meetings; surgeons have been offered this opportunity in the hope that it will stimulate their participation.

Component and Affiliate Relationships

Although two hospitals are listed as CCOP component institutions, they exist under the corporate umbrella of Oxford, which also includes a rehabilitation facility, the Carnegie Hospital. The Oxford board and senior management chose to locate the cancer program, including the CCOP, at St. Mary's Hospital, and allocate approximately $100,000 annually to the Cancer Research Program.

The merger of the West Chester and St. Mary's Hospitals more than ten years ago made Oxford a dominant medical center in the state, as well as one of the largest. Since Oxford is a tertiary medical center and most of the other hospitals are community hospitals, the level of competition between Oxford and its affiliates is relatively low; Dr. Ellens, a partner in a very busy three-physician group of family practitioners, suggested that only St. Francis Hospital competes with Oxford. In fact, Oxford considers its major competition to be the academic medical centers in two major metropolitan areas.

Oxford established affiliate relationships with the large number of small hospitals scattered throughout the region primarily because of the tradition of cooperative efforts in the state. The desire to increase the patient base for higher accrual was a secondary motivation. The relationship between Oxford and these other institutions is tenuous. Drs. Peters and Selling practice part-time at Riverside and Salem Hospitals. Dr. Manning of Collins Hospital occasionally places a patient on a protocol. However, in the vast majority of cases, a patient with cancer will be referred to Oxford if the primary physician believes a useful protocol is available. Despite Dr. Smith's efforts to educate the physician community at the affiliate hospitals, few patients from these hospitals are placed on protocol.

Although Dr. Smith says that he has had few problems with the institutional review board at Oxford, Drs. Williams and Jones complain that the institutional review board is frequently unreasonably stringent. Originally the institutional review board had two subcommittees. One concerned itself with the science of a protocol, and the second focused on human rights issues. Even Dr. Smith agreed that this framework was burdensome and caused unreasonable delays. Subsequently, about two years ago, he was able to obtain an agreement from the institutional review board that any National Cancer Institute-approved protocol would be considered scientifically valid and would be reviewed only for human rights issues. Dr. Smith estimates that most protocols are approved at a single institutional review board monthly meeting. Further, the affiliated hospitals agreed to accept the decisions of the Oxford institutional review board as binding on their institutions. As Dr. Smith describes the institutional review board, "I respect those people. Sometimes they get crazy, but then I tell them they're crazy."

The institutional review board has 11 voting members and one nonvoting member. Two of the voting members are physicians, and several are Ph.D.s with research training. Other members of the committee include two psychologists, one nurse, one attorney, one philosopher, one minister, and one retired teacher. Dr. Smith asserts that the key to moving a protocol through the institutional review board is being available at the monthly meeting to answer questions. Drs. Jones and Williams assert that the committee still occasionally concerns itself with the scientific merit of a protocol and often focuses on "trivial" human rights issues that require changing a few sentences in an informed consent document.

Organization for Cancer Control Research

All the physicians, administrators, and support staff agree that the concept of cancer prevention and control research is not clearly understood; further, Drs. Smith and Jones and Ms. Harris express concern about the cancer prevention and control credits required by each CCOP. The CCOP participants also generally feel that neither the National Cancer Institute nor the research bases provide sufficient information, guidance, or leadership concerning cancer control. Dr. Smith states that few protocols have even been offered by their cooperative group.

Although the Oxford CCOP grant proposal suggested that Oxford had substantial experience with cancer prevention and control research prior to the CCOP, Drs. Smith and Jones feel their own experience is limited. For example, Dr. Smith states that, "I'm only now getting a feel for cancer prevention and control research." Moreover, the institutional review board presents a real challenge for prevention and control protocols. Despite gaining approval from their institutional review board for a number of cancer prevention and control research projects, Drs. Smith and Jones say that many protocols closed before they could enroll patients and that others were very narrowly focused, such as providing a blood sample. Neither Dr. Smith nor Dr. Jones is certain of the cancer prevention and control protocols in which Oxford is participating; they mention a pain control protocol developed by one cooperative group and an epidemiology project by the other cooperative group. Dr. Smith also says that two projects for cancer control protocols are in development at Oxford. Dr. Peters is attempting to write a protocol concerning the screening of chemical workers for bladder cancer, while another CCOP physician is developing a smoking cessation teaching program for house staff.

Dr. Smith thinks that almost any of the protocols available could be carried out at Oxford, particularly those related to screening, pain control, and identification of psychosocial factors related to cancer issues. Dr. Jones suggests that the large-scale preventive efforts are least practical, while the patient-management protocols are most practical since they could be linked to treatment protocols. These physicians, along with Dr. Williams and Ms. Harris, express concern that the credits given for cancer prevention and control protocols are not sufficient for the work and cost involved in identifying and following the patients. Further, there is general agreement that the larger screening protocols would require the addition of more data managers and might necessitate a different data management system.

The cancer control activities include participation in: (1) the state cancer registry; (2) breast screening and management demonstration projects; (3) a tumor control center program; (4) a cancer control developmental and support program to train administrative staff; (5) a breast cancer serum collection follow-up program; and (6) American Cancer Society-sponsored smoking cessation activities. Dr. Smith also thinks that the effort to reach minorities to provide them with appropriate care has a cancer control aspect.

Many key primary physicians and administrators are interested in moving forward with cancer prevention and control research. In fact, Dr. Smith states that Ms. Johnson, the Oxford CEO, considers cancer prevention and control research a primary goal of the CCOP. The minority cancer program may develop a primary care network that may be used for cancer control research. An outpatient facility, which may provide an effective structure in which to perform some types of cancer control research, is also planned at Oxford.

Research Base Relationships

Oxford's primary CCOP research base affiliation is with a large clinical cooperative group through the University of Pennsylvania-Landhope Cancer Center. However, other physicians are linked with other cooperative groups. These research bases were chosen because of their long history of association with Oxford. However, Oxford has informed these research bases that it will choose competing protocols because of its primary affiliation through the Pennsylvania-Landhope Cancer Center. Most of the CCOP physicians regularly attend research base meetings; representative members of the CCOP support staff are also regularly given the opportunity to attend these meetings.

Drs. Smith, Jones, Lawson, and Williams feel that Oxford's relationship with the research bases is generally good. Although Oxford has no voting rights through its primary affiliation, Dr. Smith thinks the research bases are still responsive to CCOP concerns. Drs. Smith and Jones have the opportunity to design and review protocols and participate in pilot studies, and Dr. Smith sits on three research base committees. Similarly, several Oxford nurses have committee appointments.

Despite the fact that at least one afternoon at each research base meeting is devoted to cancer prevention and control, Dr. Smith suggests that the research bases "don't know how to do research in these areas." Most of the physicians agree that the most severe problem is the availability of research protocols for cancer prevention and control. Still, Dr. Smith believes that the structure and processes are in place at Oxford to perform cancer control research at such time as protocols become available. The new emphasis on cancer control research may be a vehicle by which CCOPs can gain more influence in the research bases generally.

National Cancer Institute, Division of Cancer Prevention and Control Relations

Dr. Smith has a cordial relationship with Carrie Hunter of the National Cancer Institute. He feels that, "I can call any time, and she always calls back." Dr. Hunter is also the main NCI contact for Dr. Jones and Ms. Harris. Most of the other CCOP physicians and data managers have had no contact with the National Cancer Institute. Dr. Smith speaks with Dr. Hunter at least every six months and often monthly; Ms. Harris contacts her at least monthly. The most common reason for contacting her recently relates to Oxford's probable inability to achieve the mandated 20 credits for cancer control protocols. Other issues concern data management, the state cancer registry, the minority grant, and the Children's Hospital.

The main area in which assistance and guidance is urgently sought concerns cancer prevention and control research protocols. Drs. Smith and Jones would like to see NCI take an active role in directing the participating cooperative groups to provide cancer prevention and control protocols, or they would like NCI to provide the protocols to the CCOPs directly. Further, several physicians and CCOP staff members suggest that more input must be obtained from the CCOPs concerning the credits given for patients enrolled in cancer control research protocols; generally, they assert that the credits presently proposed are unrealistically low and a barrier to accrual.

Although Drs. Smith and Jones are aware that a CCOP advisory board exists, they do not know its composition or its role in the CCOP program. More information from NCI about a range of issues and topics is generally felt to be desirable; more information or help related to cancer control protocols is considered indispensable if NCI truly wants the CCOPs to meet the cancer control credit goals.

The funding at Oxford from the CCOP program has been very useful in providing stability to a cancer research program that had been struggling for years. Additional funding would be primarily directed to the increased data management requirements resulting from cancer control research protocols.

Relationships with Community Groups

A number of voluntary community groups work with Oxford and are available for its patients. Among the groups that work with the cancer program are the American Cancer Society; Hospice, Inc.; the Ostomy Society; and the Leukemia Society. Thomas Widder, a registered nurse and the American Cancer Society representative, coordinates the Master's of Nursing program at the University of Pennsylvania and, as a friend of Dr. Miles, has long been aware of the CCOP. Shawn Owens, a registered nurse and the Hospice, Inc. representative, and Kathleen Holden, the Ostomy Society president, are aware of the availability of cancer prevention and control protocols at Oxford but are unaware of the CCOP.

Unfortunately, the general community and, more specifically, the many health-related community groups, are unaware of the CCOP at Oxford or its function. Moreover, the community representatives state that, although they personally are aware of the availability of research protocols at Oxford, most of the members of their specific groups are unaware that these exist or what they are. In contrast, Drs. Smith and Jones and other CCOP physicians believe a sizable number of the community groups are aware that protocols are available at Oxford. Many of the CCOP physicians have participated in these community groups. For example, Drs. Smith and Jones are members of the board of the American Cancer Society; Dr. Smith is the medical director of Hospice, Inc.; and Dr. Jones is on the board of the Leukemia Society. Several other CCOP physicians are involved with these or other community organizations, and nearly all the CCOP physicians refer cancer patients or their families to these groups. No community group members sit on any of the CCOP or Cancer Research Program boards or committees.

Drs. Wilson, Smith, and Jones and the administrators, Mr. Rice and Mr. Steiner, view industrial organizations in the community as a major, untapped source of potential funding for the cancer program and Oxford. Although two of the major chemical firms in the state have had a role at Oxford at the board level, these firms have contributed little to Oxford because, in the past, they have sought the prestige associated with contributions to major academic centers. Now, however, these firms are jointly funding an eight-bed unit at Oxford to perform Phase 1 trials.

Communication between the community groups and the CCOP is primarily informal. The community groups regularly send many of the CCOP physicians newsletters or announcements, and the Cancer Research Program usually sends materials to these groups as well. Still, no written materials specifically from the CCOP are sent to community groups. The community representatives are also generally unfamiliar with any specific cancer control activities performed by the CCOP or the Cancer Research Program on a regular basis. However, activities such as screening for breast and colon cancer and smoking cessation efforts have been cosponsored by the Cancer Research Program, Oxford, and some community groups.

Relationships with the Physician Community

As the dominant medical center in rural southeast Pennsylvania, Oxford has a large proportion of the physicians in the tristate area of rural Pennsylvania, Delaware, and Maryland on its staff, including all of the oncologists. It is estimated that 90 percent to 100 percent of the oncologists in the state are aware of the CCOP and the availability of National Cancer Institute-approved protocols at Oxford. Perhaps more important, the percentage of primary care physicians who are aware of the Oxford CCOP and the availability of National Cancer Institute protocols ranges from 15 percent to 40 percent. Obviously, a critical challenge is to make physicians more aware of the CCOP program and of the availability of National Cancer Institute protocols through CCOPs.

The National Cancer Institute and the research bases also need to develop protocols that include primary care physicians. More aggressive advertising of the presence and activities of CCOPs is needed at all levels — the CCOPs, research bases, and National Cancer Institute.

Questions for Discussion

1. What indicators of organizational performance would you select to assess the effectiveness of this CCOP? How effective is the CCOP on these indicators?

2. How adequate is the CCOP structure? What changes would you suggest?

3. What action must Dr. Smith take to encourage increased physician participation — in treatment protocols and in prevention and control protocols?

4. Does the availability of protocols enhance the quality of care in the community? What ethical questions arise? How might these be resolved?

5. As an increasing portion of the population is covered through some type of managed care, how will this affect the ability of CCOP to accrue patients? What are the advantages and disadvantages of managed care to a community-based trials network? What strategy will need to be developed, and/or what changes made, at the community or national level, to involve managed care in community-based clinical trials?

References

Greenwald, P., J. Cullen, and J. McKenna. 1987. "Cancer Prevention and Control: From Research to Application." *Journal of the National Cancer Institute* 79 (2): 389–400.

Kaluzny, A., J. Morrissey, and M. McKinney. 1990. "Emerging Organizational Networks: The Case of the Community Clinical Oncology Program." In *Innovations in the Organization of Health Care*, edited by S. Mick and Associates, 87–90. San Francisco: Jossey-Bass.

Kaluzny, A. D., R. Warnecke, and D. Gillings. 1992. "Assessment of the Implementation and Impact of the Community Clinical Oncology Program — Phase II." Final Report to National Cancer Institute, Cecil G. Sheps Center for Health Services Research. (Performed under contract NO1-CN-75435).

Appendix to Case 1

People Associated with the CCOP at Oxford Medical Center

Position	Name/Specialty
PI, CCOP & Minority Grant	Irving Smith, M.D. (hematology/oncology)
Co-PI	Vincent Jones, M.D.
CCOP coordinator	Susan Harris, R.N.
Investigator, PI, NSABP Grant	Timothy Lawson, M.D. (medical oncology)
President and CEO, Oxford Medical Center	Alice Johnson
Director, Cancer & Grant Program	Leslie Wilson, M.D.
Senior vice president, finance	James Rice
CCOP business manager	Max Steiner
CCOP data managers	Pamela Bell, R.N.
	Peter Simmons
Participating community physicians	Anthony Lear, M.D. Mollie Peters, M.D. Peter Selling, M.D. Bruce Williams, M.D. Stanley Doris, M.D. Laura Ruth, M.D. Elizabeth Miles, M.D. Timothy Lawson, M.D. Theodore Jane, M.D.
NCI contacts	Carrie Hunter, M.D. Joshua Miles, M.D.
American Cancer Society representative	Thomas Widder, R.N.
Hospice, Inc. representative	Shawn Ownes, R.N.
Ostomy Society President	Kathleen Holden

CASE 2

The Mt. Hope Health Council
An Emerging Public and Private Community Health Partnership

by Paul Halverson and Arnold D. Kaluzny

The local public health director, Dr. Hugh Simmons, and the president of Mt. Hope Regional Medical Center, Mr. Michael White, have been meeting regularly since Mr. White became the president of the hospital three years ago. Mr. White has long held that the hospital must move beyond its traditional focus on acute care and become more involved with the health of the larger community. Since Dr. Simmons and Mr. White have been meeting, the health department and the hospital have initiated several joint efforts. Most of the efforts have centered around health promotion programs, but a recent effort has resulted in the joint funding and operation of a residency program for two preventive medicine fellows.

Dr. Simmons and Mr. White are also aware that rapidly rising health insurance premiums have frustrated the already difficult economic conditions faced by many employers in the Mt. Hope area. Mt. Hope workers have felt the effect of rising health care costs through lower wages, reductions or eliminations in employer-paid medical benefits, and business closures. Concerns located outside of Mt. Hope own six of the 14 manufacturing plants that employ 200 or more workers. The plant managers from these firms have incorporated various cost-containment strategies in their health care purchasing decisions. Mr. Larry Johnson, the general manager for Minnesota Electronics (2,000 employees in Mt. Hope) was recently elected to head the Mt. Hope Employer Coalition. This organization was formed primarily to pressure health provider organizations to lower costs and increase accountability for employer investment in health care. The coalition hired the university's Health Research Center to study health costs and outcomes in their community and to make recommendations for reducing costs and increasing quality. While all of the large employers in the area are members of the coalition, the small employers are represented by a contingent of Mt. Hope Area Chamber of Commerce members that serve on the coalition's board of directors. By design, no health care provider has been invited or allowed to participate. This policy has caused more than a moderate degree of tension for the normally cooperative and friendly Mt. Hope, Minnesota community. The board of directors has recently announced the appointment of Malcom Berkstrom, M.D., Ph.D., as the president of the coalition. Dr. Berkstrom comes to Mt. Hope out of his recent retirement from a large biotechnology firm in Chicago.

The managed care environment for Mt. Hope continues to be an anomaly for communities of this size. For example, less than 10 percent of the individuals in Mt. Hope with some form of private health insurance are enrolled in managed care plans. This low degree of market penetration exists in part due to the efforts of the Hope Clinic to resist any form of managed care. Despite formal requests from the many employers in the area, the Hope Clinic has been successful in preserving its exclusively fee-for-service reimbursement arrangements. Each of the hospitals and most other physicians, however, participate in the managed care plans popular in other areas of the region.

At their last quarterly medical staff meeting, Mt. Hope Regional Medical Center announced the results of their strategic planning efforts. The strategic plan approved by the hospital board of directors calls for the creation of a new physician-hospital organization (PHO) and an aggressive plan for developing managed care capacity. The long-range plan is to develop a new entity that would be owned jointly by the medical center, a yet-to-be-formed physician company, the county health department, and an insurance company. The format of the organization is similar to many of the existing PHO models, with the exception of adding the public health department. The medical center executive staff is convinced that managed care organizations will continue their movement toward more population-based service delivery approaches and, as such, any new health system needs to contain experience and expertise in public health. The public health department offers both the capacity and the expertise to serve populations with which the hospital has little experience, along with the necessary experience in assessment and policy development.

In connection with the new strategic plan, Mt. Hope Regional announced the acquisition of a new, 40-physician primary care group known as Health Partners. Under the purchase agreement, Health Partners will remain a separate physician group whose assets are owned by the medical center, and the group will add an additional 20 physicians in the next two years. The announcement has created a furor among physicians at the Hope Clinic, who have practiced primarily at the medical center. The Hope Clinic physicians have long resisted any arrangement with hospitals on ideological grounds, claiming nonphysician involvement in their practice would ultimately lead to diminished autonomy and control over their practice.

Meanwhile, heated discussions at county commission meetings and in the press have centered around the nearly $50 million facility replacement request by Hope County Hospital. The county commissioners have fielded much of the controversy, since they act as the hospital board and must keep all meetings open to the public. The hospital is over 100 years old and is in obvious need of replacement or major renovation. Although the facility is available to serve all patients, Medicaid and indigent patients account for almost 70 percent of the payer mix for the hospital. The county's subsidization of the facility has averaged $1.2 million over the last five years. The recent resignation of the hospital's administrator shocked the county commissioners, who had recently increased the administrator's salary to $50,000. Six different administrators have headed the hospital in the last ten years.

The local social services director recently released expenditure records showing that the county's social service board had spent over $2 million for medical services provided outside of the county. This figure, along with recently released statistics indicating Mt. Hope has the state's worst infant mortality rate, has created general alarm in the community. Access to physician care by Medicaid and indigent patients is very restricted. Most physicians either do not accept or greatly limit their involvement with low-income patients. Stating concerns over low payment and increased liability, the Hope Clinic last year announced their providers would no longer participate in the care of nonemergent Medicaid or indigent patients. The only obstetric care available to Medicaid and indigent patients is provided at Hope County Hospital, where three obstetrics/gynecology residents rotate as part of their training. Recent attempts to initiate nurse-midwife services at both Mt. Hope hospitals have been scuttled because of the refusal of physicians to provide credentials and clinical support for midwifes. Grant funds available from the state health department to the local health department for improving access to prenatal care and obstetrical case management have gone unused because of the active opposition of the county medical society to health department involvement in providing direct clinical care to patients.

Mt. Hope Health Council

Perplexed and frustrated by the problems of access for the indigent, high infant mortality, and concerns over the potential activities of the employer coalition, Dr. Simmons and Mr. White invited the administrator of the county hospital, directors of social services, mental health, nursing homes, home health, the community health center, and two administrators from the medical groups to a breakfast meeting at the medical center. While each of the administrators had lived within the community for a number of years, there were a number of participants at the meeting who had not met each other before. The meeting was primarily designed as a get-acquainted meeting to determine if there was enough common interest in formalizing the group with a goal of improving the health of the community. The meeting went exceptionally well, and the group decided unanimously to meet on a regular basis as the Mt. Hope Health Council. The two specific issues on which the group decided to concentrate were access to medical care (especially prenatal and obstetrical care), and the development of a community health assessment (especially related to appropriate measurement of health status). In addition, Dr. Berkstrom from the employer coalition was invited to become a member of the council.

Dr. Simmons was elected as the chair and Mr. White as the vice chair of the Mt. Hope Health Council. Mr. White volunteered his vice president of planning and marketing and his staff to provide assistance for the council. Two task forces were established to address the two priorities the Council had established. Mr. White chaired the task force on access, and Dr. Simmons the task force on community health.

Access Task Force Activities

Mr. White charged his task force to: (1) identify the extent of the problem related to access to health care for indigent and other at-risk people; (2) identify specific barriers to access and the principal causes of these barriers; (3) identify long-range and short-range opportunities to improve access to health care; and (4) recommend a course of action to the council for implementation. In consultation with the council, the committee appointed 19 individuals to serve on the task force, including representatives from government, business, the university, and the major health care and social services providers within the county. Table 1 shows the 19 appointees to the task force.

Table 1. Appointees to the Task Force on Access

1. Vice president for community health of Mt. Hope Regional Medical Center
2. Chief of staff from Hope County Hospital
3. Director of social services of Hope County Hospital
4. Director of the county department of social services
5. Medical director of the county health department
6. Director of the Hope Regional Homecare Company
7. Director of Tender Home (nursing home)
8. Executive director of the Hope County United Way
9. Director of the Salvation Army homeless shelter
10. Director of adult health from the county health department
11. President of the Hope County Medical Society
12. Administrator of the Health Partners clinic
13. Medical director of the Hope Clinic
14. Professor from the School of Public Health
15. President of the Chamber of Commerce (a banker)
16. School superintendent
17. Vice mayor of the city
18. County administrator
19. President of the Junior League

Most of the appointees to the task force were eager to serve, although a few needed some persuasion to see the value in their participation. The presidents of the Chamber of Commerce and the Junior League were completely unaware of any problems with access to medical care in the community. They were also surprised to learn that Mt. Hope even had a homeless shelter. The president of the medical society knew only that the task force was being formed to allow the health department to operate a personal care clinic, and begrudgingly accepted his appointment just to make sure such a plan was not seriously considered. The medical director of the Hope Clinic knew that the other appointees might give the task force significant latitude for action. He resigned himself to serving on it to help shape its actions, in spite of the liberal ideas he knew that he would have to fight.

After reviewing data gathered by a subcommittee of the task force on access to health care, the task force began to realize as a group the serious problems existing within their county. They learned that over 30 percent of the population had no type of health insurance, and that projected plant closures threatened to increase that number. The task force discovered that low-income people were not the only individuals without health insurance. Data indicated that many self-employed, temporary, and part-time workers, as well as individuals with preexisting medical conditions, lacked adequate health insurance.

The task force recognized the lack of health insurance as a major barrier to receiving care in their community. They learned that because of a serious shortage of physicians in their community, health services were often limited or completely unavailable to uninsured individuals. Data revealed that if an uninsured woman became pregnant, she would have to travel over an hour to the next county to receive prenatal care, since no physician in the local community provided obstetrical care to patients without insurance (except by special arrangement). The task force discovered that access to clinical preventive services was also extremely limited for the uninsured. Few primary care physicians granted office or clinic visits to individuals without insurance. Consequently, many serious health problems, which could have been prevented or treated earlier in a much less costly setting, were treated in local emergency rooms.

Many of the task force members now confronted for the first time the major, communitywide implications stemming from inadequate access to health care. Task force members recognized a self-perpetuating cycle of declining community health, characterized by: (1) physician groups and clinics resisting providing preventive and primary care services to the uninsured; (2) hospitals providing costly acute care services to a population often unable to pay for such services; (3) hospitals recouping the costs associated with caring for the uninsured by raising the fees charged to paying patients; (4) insurance companies responded to rising hospital fees by increasing the health insurance premiums paid by businesses; (5) employers responding to increasing health insurance premiums by reducing or eliminating benefits, eliminating jobs, or ceasing operations. Even the budget-minded county administrator began to acknowledge the problem when it was pointed out that uninsured individuals are more likely to experience more health problems, resulting in lost wage earnings, lower employment levels and, consequently, fewer dollars paid in taxes. Aside from the Hope Clinic medical director, who questioned the accuracy of the data, the task force overwhelmingly accepted the report describing the extent of inadequate health care access in the county.

The task force recognized that a variety of factors within the county discouraged or prevented access to health care services for those individuals without adequate health insurance. They identified these factors and ranked them by the frequency in which they occurred, as shown in Table 2. Interviews with providers revealed that at least some of these barriers to care stemmed from the attitudes and practices of providers, which are shown in Table 3. In addition to those reported by providers, the task force identified other causes of the barriers to access which are shown in Table 4. The task force realized that there were many more reasons for the barriers to care, but settled on those listed as the primary determinants.

Table 2. Barriers to Health Care Access, by Frequency

1. Inability to obtain a physician appointment for care
2. Lack of transportation to medical care facilities
3. Lack of childcare during appointment
4. Loss of earnings during appointment
5. Inability to take time off from work for fear of losing job
6. Excessive wait time for an appointment
7. Hostile attitude of nurses and physicians
8. Language barrier
9. Inability to read
10. Physical barriers to access to medical facilities
11. Lack of knowledge regarding need for care

Table 3. Reasons for Barriers to Access, Reported by Providers

1. Fear of increased malpractice risk
2. Providers' past experience with lack of compliance, particularly in taking medications
3. Lack of waiting room space (especially for large families)
4. Incompatibility with existing clientele
5. Language barriers

Table 4. Other Reasons for Barriers to Access

1. Shortage of physicians
2. Lack of interest by physicians in caring for indigent patients
3. Lack of public transportation
4. Illiteracy
5. Unemployment
6. Low-wage, low-skill employment
7. Poverty
8. Provider participation in integrated systems of care, which provide services only to patients enrolled in the system
9. Inconvenient locations and hours of operation

The task force discussed long-range solutions, and considered the following:

1. Lowering the unemployment rates
2. Increasing the socioeconomic status of area residents
3. Improving the health status of area residents
4. Increasing consumers' knowledge of the health system
5. Increasing the supply of health providers (including physician extenders)
6. Offering incentives for providers to keep patients healthy (not fee-for-service)
7. Developing a patient-centered health system

A great deal of debate ensued over many meetings as to the proper long-range solutions, but the task force voted these seven solutions as being primary to improving access to health care. Many of the health professionals on the task force were initially very resistant to acknowledging the effect of unemployment or socioeconomic factors on health care access. Presentations by the public health professionals helped to elucidate these issues and bring consensus to the group on this issue.

The task force also identified short-term strategies for improving access to health care, which included

1. Developing a communitywide physician recruitment effort (independent of the physician groups that resisted bringing new physicians to town)
2. Developing a satellite office to the existing community health center

3. Contracting for obstetrics/gynecology physician services and nurse-midwife services

4. Developing a primary care clinic as a joint venture between agencies

5. Determining the feasibility of developing a community managed care program (in which all community health providers would participate)

6. Developing school-based primary care clinics

7. Developing primary care clinics at major employer locations

8. Determining the feasibility of requiring all physicians who have hospital privileges (at both hospitals) to provide coverage for indigent patients on an equal basis

9. Considering the privatization of the county hospital and public health department and shifting resources for redundant services to pay for indigent care

10. Considering the development of a managed care program administered jointly by the county hospital and the county public health department

The task force considered each of the ten short-term options carefully, and after much debate advanced two proposals to the council for immediate implementation: the communitywide physician recruitment effort and the joint-venture primary care clinic.

Task Force on Community Health

Dr. Simmons appointed a 20-member task force that included health and social services providers representatives from government, business, law enforcement, and the media. Table 5 shows the appointees to this task force. The first order of business for the task force was to become oriented with the principles of public health and the core functions that constitute public health responsibility. The professor from the School of Public Health was a good resource as the members of the task force began to understand the scope of what public health entails. They agreed that the mission of the task force was to evaluate, and recommend strategies that contribute to the improvement of, the health for the Mt. Hope community.

The task force set as their first goal an evaluation of the current health status of the community by conducting a community health assessment. While the health department had been conducting something called a "community diagnosis" for years, Dr. Simmons acknowledged that it had been primarily an internal process of comparing secondary data as a requirement of the state health department. The hospital administrators claimed they had also been performing "community assessment" activities as part of their annual strategic planning processes, but also acknowledged the rather narrow focus of this

Table 5. Appointees to the Community Health Task Force

1. County administrator
2. City manager
3. County board chairman
4. Mayor
5. President of the Chamber of Commerce
6. Administrator of Hope County Hospital
7. Administrator of Mt. Hope Regional Medical Center
8. President of the Hope County Medical Society
9. Director of the county department of social services
10. Administrator of the Hope Clinic
11. Vice president for community health at Mt. Hope Regional Medical Center
12. Local newspaper editor
13. President of the Hope County United Way
14. Administrator of the community mental health center
15. School superintendent
16. Police chief
17. Sheriff
18. Director of public safety
19. County clerk
20. Faculty member from the School of Public Health

activity related to acute care. The task force agreed that the process needed to be much more inclusive and comprehensive than what had previously been done. The task force agreed that they would ask the School of Public Health to make a recommendation on how they should conduct the community assessment.

The hospital administrators indicated that they had been approached by many different consulting groups interested in conducting a community assessment. Dr. Simmons mentioned the assessment models developed by the Centers for Disease Control and Prevention, including PATCH (Planned Approach to Community Health) and APEX-PH (Assessment Protocol for Excellence in Public Health). The School of Public Health's Center for Public Health Practice recommended an assessment method that included secondary data analysis; primary data gathering through surveys, focus groups, and key informant interviews; and the use of a community priority-setting process. The school further indicated that the assessment process should be developed in an open and inclusive manner with the community.

The community health task force decided that conducting a community assessment was an essential first step for their effort, and one that would require a great deal of community support and resources. In recognition of this, they decided that they would recommend to the council that the community health task force take responsibility for conducting a comprehensive community assessment. They decided to request that the council sanction this activity and find funding to support the consulting fees and publication costs. In addition, the task force decided that each of its members should seek the endorsement of each of their respective organizations as a means of communicating the importance of this effort.

Population and Unemployment

Mt. Hope is located in a community of nearly 200,000 people. While the City of Mt. Hope includes many light manufacturing industries and a growing service sector, the surrounding counties and population areas are considerably smaller and rural.

Unemployment rates for Mt. Hope have been well below the state average for nearly 50 years, owing primarily to the success of manufacturing operations oriented toward the defense industry. Recent changes in governmental defense spending, however, have prompted the announcement of plant closures in Mt. Hope that will result in the layoff of over 5,000 plant workers, plus an unknown number of service and support positions. The closures are scheduled to take place in three months.

An excerpt from the 1990 census for Mt. Hope appears in Table 6. Of particular note is the growing elderly population and the increasing number of people between the ages of 12 and 24. While the community growth rate has been approximately 5 percent each year for the past ten years, roughly 3 percent is attributable to new people moving to the area. Another interesting fact is that over 40 percent of the families in Mt. Hope have lived in the community for 20 years or more. There is a strong sense of family and community.

Table 6. Census Data for Mt. Hope

	1990	*1980*
Population	194,110	169,742
Percent under 5 years	6.5	7.2
Percent 5 to 17 years	16.4	13.9
Percent 18 to 64 years	62.9	67.7
Percent 65 years and older	14.2	11.2
Percent that moved during last 10 years	32.1	29.8
Median household income (adjusted)	$27,518	$28,119
Median members per household	3	3
Unemployment rate	3.7	2.8

Government

Mt. Hope enjoys a long heritage of strong but conservative local government. Mt. Hope operates under a mayor-council-manager form of government. The mayor serves a five-year term and cannot be reelected. The city council consists of six council members, elected to three-year terms for a maximum of three terms. The city manager is appointed by the mayor and serves at the pleasure of the city council. With only two other towns of limited size in its jurisdiction, Hope County government largely serves the needs of the Mt. Hope community. The county is governed by a nine-person board of commissioners. The commissioners serve four-year terms and can be reelected without limitation. The chairman of the board of commissioners is selected annually by a vote of the commission. The county administrator is appointed by the board of commissioners to a five-year renewable term. All elected offices require prior residency within the city or the county for a minimum of ten years. The city manager has been on the job for two years, and the county administrator for 22 years. The newest elected officials (three city councilmen and two county commissioners) have been in office for nine months. The new officeholders were elected after having publicly sworn to cut taxes and decrease government bureaucracy.

Health Resources

The county is served by two hospitals, 280 physicians, 82 dentists, a community health center, a county health department, five nursing homes, and five home health agencies.

Hospitals

The two hospitals include Mt. Hope Regional Medical Center and Hope County Hospital. Mt. Hope Regional is a 380-bed teaching hospital owned by a non-profit integrated health system in Minneapolis. Hope County Hospital is an 82-bed, county-operated acute care facility. The hospitals are located two blocks from each other in Mt. Hope. Table 7 lists operating statistics from the 1995 AHA guide.

Table 7. 1995 Hospital Statistics

	Mt. Hope Regional	*Hope County Hospital*
Beds	380	82
Outpatient visits	53,476	2,346
Average daily census	212	61
1993 discharges	26,743	949
Births	1,240	153
Deaths	458	105
Average length of stay (days)	13.8	19.2

Physicians
Table 8 lists physician specialties and median ages. Nearly 100 physicians practice together in the Hope Clinic group practice. The new, 40-physician Health Partners group consists solely of primary care physicians. The remaining physicians practice solo or in pairs. Mt. Hope physicians have a median length of time in the community of 12 years. Thirty percent of the physicians are doctors of osteopathy. Eighty-two percent are board-certified or eligible.

Dentists
One group practice of 20 dentists operates within the community. A dental health maintenance organization in Minneapolis owns this practice. Five dentists work full-time in the public health dental clinics. The remaining dentists practice alone or in pairs.

Community Health Center
The federally qualified community health center is located in the southern part of the city, near the small town of Mt. Pleasant. The community health center contracts with many different physicians for part-time coverage. Over the last two years, the center's costs were 10 percent lower than the maximum reimbursement levels allowed for federal funding.

Table 8. Physician Demographics

Specialty	Number	Median Age
Anesthesiology	5	48
Child psychiatry	11	46
Diagnostic radiology	6	43
Family practice	9	52
Gastroenterology	5	42
General practice	31	51
General surgery	23	47
Internal medicine	43	52
Obstetrics/gyn.	24	39
Ophthalmology	11	48
Orthopedic surgery	13	42
Otolaryngology	3	58
Pathology/anatomy	12	63
Pediatrics	24	54
Psychiatry	8	42
Radiology	6	37
Urology	9	52
Inactive	37	69
Total	280	51

Health Department

The city and county jointly operate the local health department. The department functions under the leadership of a doctorally prepared public health director, who reports to a city-county board of health. Two city council members and two county commissioners sit on the board of health, in addition to the health director who serves as the vice chair. The department consists of 110 employees working at three separate sites. Clinical services provided by the health department are limited by county ordinance to sexually transmitted diseases, immunizations, health screening, and infectious disease control and treatment. County ordinance also authorizes a home health division within the department, which consists of 20 nurses. In addition to clinical services, the health department is responsible for vital records, restaurant inspections, environmental health, and "all other population-based services deemed necessary and important to the health of the public." In providing both clinical and population-based services, the department collects and analyzes a broad array of health statistics for its jurisdiction. Table 9 presents some of these statistics.

Table 9. Selected Health Statistics

Live births (1995)	1,393
Total infant deaths	102
Fetal deaths	56
Deaths under 28 days	27
Deaths under 1 year	19
Noninfant deaths by major causes (1995)	
Total	1,145
Infections	13
Neoplasms	354
Diabetes	41
Cardiovascular	367
Cerebrovascular	85
Chronic obstructive	32
Motor vehicle accidents	31
Other accidents	37
Suicide	7
Homicide	0
Other	178
Risk factor prevalence (1992)	
Percent with high blood pressure	31.2
Percent with high cholesterol	37.9
Percent smokers	17.3

Nursing Homes

All five of the nursing homes in the county are certified for both Medicare and Medicaid patients. The Medicaid reimbursement for nursing home residents in the county is nearly 80 percent. Each of the nursing homes is fully occupied at least 90 percent of the year, and most have extensive waiting lists for beds. One of the facilities is nonprofit, and one is operated by the county. The other three are proprietary institutions.

Home Health

The home health agencies in the county include two agencies with federally certified hospice benefits, and three with durable medical equipment subsidiaries. Of the five agencies, the health department operates one, each of the hospitals operates one, one is operated by the local Lutheran church, and the fifth agency is owned and operated by Acme Pharmaceuticals of North Carolina. Each of the home health agencies is Medicare certified.

Questions for Discussion

1. What action should the Mt. Hope Health Council take with the recommendations of the task forces?

2. What advantages and barriers are created by the divergent interests involved in problem-solving activities?

3. What is the appropriate balance between the two council priorities — access and community health — in terms of priorities and actions?

Acquiring Group Practices for a Vertically Integrated Health System

by Paul F. Primeau

Gramercy Health System has acquired three group practices since October 1984. Many benefits, both expected and unexpected, have accrued to Gramercy as a result of these acquisitions. Each of the three groups has contributed to the system in different ways. Careful planning of acquisition transition into the health system has been important to maintaining positive employee relations and to realizing anticipated benefits quickly. Gramercy's experience in assimilating three different types of groups can be helpful to other health systems considering acquisitions of physician group practices.

Gramercy, a Vertically Integrated System

For Gramercy, a growing, vertically integrated health system, capturing market share through an expanding medical staff has been an important strategy. Group practice acquisition is a rapid way to increase the size of the medical staff and system market share.

Hospitals

Gramercy Health System has a total of five hospitals. At the center of the system is a 939-bed tertiary hospital in an urban location. The tertiary hospital has a closed-staff, 900-physician group practice, Harvest Health. Besides the urban hospital, there are two suburban acute care hospitals and two specialty hospitals, one for chemical dependency and one for psychiatric treatment.

With almost 2,000 hospital beds to fill and lengths of stay declining, Gramercy has significant financial risk. Lengths of stay have decreased in part because of new technology that allows what used to be inpatient procedures to be performed as outpatient services. Also, changing reimbursement methods (e.g., DRGs and other methods of managed care) provide financial incentives for shorter lengths of stay. Thus, to use its 2,000 hospital beds fully, Gramercy is interested in expanding the size of its medical staff to capture greater market share.

Medical Staff Configuration

Within the health system, there are two group practice organizations and approximately 1,500 physicians in private practice.

The medical staff at the psychiatric and suburban acute care hospitals consist principally of private practice physicians. During the last six years, a significant number of group practice physicians have been appointed to these hospital staffs.

The larger of the two group practices, Harvest Health, has approximately 900 physicians. Harvest Health accepts both fee-for-service and managed care patients. The managed care segment of the practice now accounts for approximately 40 percent of its revenue. The smaller group practice, Gladstone Medical Group, comprises approximately 150 physicians. This group practices as a staff model for the system's HMO.

The three group practices Gramercy has acquired have been integrated, for governance and operations purposes, into Harvest Health.

Managed Care Organization

The Gramercy Health System has a 450,000-member HMO. The HMO has contracts with independent practice association (IPA) networks as well as with group practices. Local performance by IPA networks is similar to industrywide experiences, in that the local IPAs have had difficulty in successfully managing care in a capitated environment. Thus, the HMO relies upon Gramercy's group practices to absorb new members. Approximately 325,000 of the 450,000 HMO members are assigned to Harvest Health and Gladstone Medical Group.

Diversified Services

Gramercy also has a number of diversified services, which require feeder networks to assure economic viability. Diversified services include transcription, pharmacy, dialysis, and home health services and optometry product lines.

The Practices Gramercy Acquired

There are many reasons to acquire group practices. This section describes Gramercy's purposes for acquiring three such practices. As one organization undertakes the acquisition of another, the benefits to both organizations need to be understood.

Faculty Associates

A multispecialty not-for-profit group practice, Faculty Associates, was established in the late 1970s. The formation of the group was the result of a medical school's administration deciding that it could no longer provide professional staffing and training programs for busy County Hospital. A faction of the medical school faculty decided to form a new group practice to staff the hospital.

Faculty Associates was formed to conduct research and provide accessible ambulatory care for the community, as well as to provide inpatient specialty services to County Hospital. Because of these purposes, the group was successful in obtaining not-for-profit status, under Section 501(c)(3) of the Internal Revenue Service Code.

Faculty Associates comprised approximately 30 physicians. Most were part-time group members. The group was fortunate in that research funding from various studies at County Hospital had generated significant surpluses in the past. These surpluses provided the initial capitalization required to purchase land and construct an 8,500-square-foot ambulatory care center without any debt. Faculty Associates also entered into agreements with County Hospital for inpatient services, which guaranteed the income of three of the group members.

Regrettably, after separation from the medical school, the ability of the new group practice to compete successfully for research funding was diminished. Thus, the group had to rely on clinical revenues for funding. Some of the original members dropped out of the group, since the original purpose of the organization was changing to cope with a new economic environment. The group also realized that, to capture the necessary market share, it would have to become involved with managed care. Thus, it entered into a contract with an HMO. The HMO grew quickly and soon accounted for approximately 60 percent of the group's revenue.

Despite a reasonable revenue stream from ambulatory care services, Faculty Associates was depleting its working capital. Income distribution for group members was based on former earnings as university faculty and not dependent on clinical productivity. The group's future financial viability was dependent solely on its ability to generate patient care revenues.

By early 1987, the group had reduced its size to seven full-time and nine part-time physicians. The monthly cash flow was approximately $40,000 short of requirements. Estimates were made, and the group members realized that they needed either to become part of a larger health care system, or to redeploy their assets for other charitable purposes, since they were operating as a not-for-profit organization. Any redeployment of assets would require approval of the state attorney general because of the group's not-for-profit status.

The group chose to look for an affiliation with a larger system, to take advantage of highly developed management systems and economies of scale, and to gain access to new sources of patients. In July 1987, Gramercy Health System acquired the assets of Faculty Associates. Gramercy chose to merge the operations of Faculty Associates with those of Harvest Health, as Gramercy's strategic plan called for an ambulatory primary care medical center in the community in which Faculty Associates was located. Faculty Associates' facility was relatively new and debt free and well suited to this purpose. The Faculty Associates internists and pediatricians were well trained and experienced and had demonstrated compatibility with group practice membership.

The newly expanded Harvest Health retained five of Faculty Associates' full-time and three of its part-time physicians. For system compatibility, business and clinical systems were converted to those used at all other Gramercy medical centers.

Physician income for the Faculty Associates doctors joining Harvest Health was maintained at former levels, with a required productivity level set. It was agreed that physician patient revenue for the remainder of 1987 would be used to determine 1988 salary levels.

The merger of this multispecialty, not-for-profit professional corporation with Gramercy Health System has been successful. Both Faculty Associates and Harvest Health understood the business plan for revamping operations before the merger. All support staff were retained or chose to decline offered positions. Faculty Associates suffered a deficit in the first six months of operation after expansion. However, by the third year, its positive contribution was significant. Figure 1 displays the contribution for the three years after the merger.

Practice Partners

Practice Partners, a for-profit multispecialty group practice, was formed in the 1950s to provide accessible ambulatory care in a southern suburban area. By October 1984, the group had grown to more than 30 physicians and two locations. The group had concentrated its efforts at developing significant market share through entering into a managed care contract with a national HMO. The proportion of revenue attributable to the HMO had increased to 60 percent. The HMO membership assigned was over 25,000 members.

Practice Partners had completed a strategic planning process and realized the following:

Figure 1. Faculty Associates Financial Performance

	1987	1988	1989
Gross contribution	($144,400)	$143,700	$751,100
Overhead	$91,100	$155,800	$176,000
Net contribution	($235,500)	($12,100)	$575,200

- The majority of revenue in the future would result from managed care contracts.

- The present national HMO that accounted for 60 percent of the group's revenue had undergone two reorganizations already and was likely to go through others. The principal model for the HMO's delivery system was through IPAs.

- Local hospitals and health systems were interested in acquiring group practices. This presented an opportunity for group members to realize equity from the practice before reaching retirement age.

- Local health systems were likely to enter the southern suburban markets with ambulatory care programs and to compete for market share if they were unable to acquire an existing group. At least three health systems were interested in having ambulatory care programs in the service area.

- The largest freestanding group practices in the metropolitan area had recently sold their practices to health systems.

- Practice Partners represented a significant opportunity to move hospital admissions for acute and tertiary care, accounting for approximately 2,500 annual inpatient admissions. Present admission patterns were to a freestanding acute care community hospital for primary and secondary care, and to one of four other institutions for tertiary care.

As a result of the strategic planning process, Practice Partners decided that they would approach the three largest health systems and offer them the opportunity to acquire the group practice. All three organizations were interested, and Practice Partners had to select one of the organizations. In two instances, Gramercy and one other, the economic considerations were identical and superior to the third option. The partnership made the decision to affiliate with Gramercy Health System because of two factors. The first was that Gramercy had a tradition of group practice. The system had 70 years of experience with group practice. The other organization had a private medical staff and medical school faculty plan. Practice Partners felt that Gramercy's group practice model was most compatible with their culture. The second factor in selecting merger with the Gramercy Health System was that Gramercy offered access to its 450,000 HMO members. In view of the organizational instability of Practice Partners' present HMO arrangement, they felt that affiliation with Gramercy would offer the most promise of assuring future patient revenues. The other system did not have an integrated managed care vehicle.

Gramercy, for its part, evaluated the opportunity to acquire Practice Partners in comparison to building a similar group practice of 30 physicians de novo. Based on previous experience in the northeast suburbs, Gramercy could simulate the cost of developing a 30-physician group. At the offer price for

Practice Partners, it was less costly to acquire the group. It was also clear that the time frame for de novo site development and physician recruitment would probably be five years. Immediate benefits would be possible through practice acquisition. Lastly, Medicare had just introduced the DRG payment methodology, and Gramercy's concern for maintaining high occupancy at its tertiary care hospital was paramount. Thus, Gramercy acquired Practice Partners.

First Care

First Care, a family practice group of six physicians, served as a faculty to an 18-resident training program at Hillside Hospital, a suburban hospital that competes with one of Gramercy's suburban hospitals.

The partner who owned 84 percent of the stock in First Care had several reasons for wanting to affiliate with an integrated health system. A few of these were:

- A vision of developing a network of several family practice training sites. Hillside Hospital was unlikely to allow development of this concept
- The ability to realize the goodwill value of the practice
- The need to take on a new challenge

Gramercy Health System was interested in acquiring First Care and in establishing a family practice training program at one of Gramercy's suburban hospitals. In February 1988, five of the six First Care physicians joined Gramercy. Three ambulatory medical care centers were opened in the summer of 1988. By September 1988, a family practice residency program was approved at one of Gramercy's suburban hospitals. The residency review committee approved 18 positions.

This was an important accomplishment for Gramercy since its suburban hospital previously had no residency programs. The new residency program promised to be a source of future medical staff. Also important is the fact that, despite the Gramercy Health System having residencies in almost all specialties, it had had none in family practice. As an integrated health system, Gramercy recognized the need for and difficulty of recruiting primary care physicians. The family practice training program would assist in meeting future primary care physician recruitment requirements.

The Benefits of Group Practice Acquisition

Gramercy Health System has reaped many benefits through its acquisition of Faculty Associates, Practice Partners, and First Care.

Hospital Admissions

Hospital admissions are a major reason for acquiring group practices. The 30 physicians who came from Faculty Associates generate 2,500 annual hospital admissions for Gramercy, valued at approximately $15 million. These admissions prior to 1984 were directed to other health systems and have now been shifted into Gramercy hospitals. For the system hospital in the southern region, this has made a significant positive contribution to profitability.

The family practice physicians from First Care have contributed to the success of Gramercy's eastside acute care hospital. The family practice residency program now accounts for approximately 600 admissions annually. Before these admissions were available, the hospital was operating at a deficit. It now has a favorable contribution. The hospital attributes the turnaround of its financial performance to the establishment of the family practice training program.

The Value of Referral Business

Gramercy recently completed a study to determine the financial value of new fee-for-service patients that entered the system through an ambulatory care medical center. The study indicated that, for each dollar of revenue generated on-site, four additional dollars were generated at other locations in the system during the same calendar year.

The value of managed care business to Gramercy is much easier to determine, since the capitation dollars are distributed to the various divisions that provide services for members. Each new member assigned to Faculty Associates, Harvest Health, and Gladstone Medical Group, adds approximately $1,200 of revenue annually. The three acquired group practices now have over 33,000 assigned HMO members.

Access Points for Market Share

As Gramercy has added group practices to its system, it has improved its accessibility to potential patients. The system now has over 30 ambulatory care locations operated by the group practices throughout the metropolitan area. This delivery system is attractive to potential HMO members and fee-for-service patients. Much of the growth in HMO membership is attributable to accessible medical centers.

Barriers to Integration

Gramercy has encountered a number of barriers to easy integration as it assimilated each of the three group practices into the system. The first is that physicians in the acquired group practices have comfort levels with existing relationships. These relationships include those with local hospital administration, specialty consultants and referral patterns, durable medical equipment suppliers, and various medical and surgical suppliers. To the extent that an integrated system offers similar or alternative services, these comfortable relationships will be altered.

A second area of conflict has been the timetable for integration of services within the system. At least one of the groups felt that the reason it was acquired was because it was well operated. It expected the system to adopt the group's methods of operation. A way to avoid this pitfall is to prepare a detailed operating plan for transition into the system.

The third barrier to smooth transition Gramercy experienced occurred in the case of smaller group practices or practices whose founding member was the chief medical officer. This was that the small practice had little understanding of the dynamics of decision making in a very large organization that values consensus. The smaller the group, the greater the likelihood of this problem.

Hints for a Smooth Integration Process

The process of integrating a group practice into a larger organization requires careful planning. The most important function to be performed is assignment of a project team, with a physician and an administrative leader from the acquiring organization, who have final decision-making authority to resolve operational problems expediently. A human resource organizational development consultant should also be on the project team if available.

When possible, a respected manager or physician from the acquiring organization should join the newly acquired group and work side by side with the staff. This begins the informal cultural transformation that is necessary for long-term success. It also provides an advocate for the system to help solve problems while they are minor.

The last tip is to leave as many as possible of the group practice's operational systems and procedures unchanged for as long as possible. This is difficult for a large system, but important to the acquired organization.

Closing Statement

As health systems acquire physician group practices, careful planning is necessary to assure that the expected benefits are realized quickly. The planning process starts during the merger feasibility phase of the relationship. It is important to develop a detailed transition plan early in the relationship. The vertically integrated health system usually has a number of objectives to accomplish, including increasing admissions, generating new referrals for other physicians already in the system, expanding managed care market share, starting new hospital or ambulatory programs, and feeding new referral business to diversified services divisions.

Gramercy Health System has successfully acquired three group practices and achieved many benefits. The major benefits include:

- An increase of over 3,500 annual admissions formerly going to competing hospitals
- Approval of a family practice training program by the residency review committee in less than a year
- Six new ambulatory medical center locations
- Over 30,000 new HMO members using the health system resources
- Over 40 new physicians added to the group practice

Clearly, the acquisition of physician group practices has increased market share for this vertically integrated health system.

Questions for Discussion

1. In order of importance, what are the reasons that a health system would want to acquire primary care group practices?
2. What are the major problems that the system could expect to encounter when acquiring group practices?
3. If you were in charge, what strategies would you employ to minimize the effect of these problems?
4. One of the group practices utilized surplus funds from research programs to establish a clinical program and new building.
5. Was this appropriate? If not, why not?
6. What information and data would you want to collect about a group practice that you were possibly interested in acquiring?

CASE 4

Linking Up with the Big City

by Lane Savitch

In May 1993, the leadership of River Valley Community Hospital held its annual retreat to contemplate the future. The leadership consisted of three elected
hospital district commissioners; the hospital administrator, Earl Young; three
assistant administrators; the five members of the medical staff executive committee, including Dr. Jo Baker, president of the Enterprise Medical Group; the
hospital medical director; the hospital attorney; and an outside facilitator. Of
the six physicians present, five were members of the Enterprise Medical Group,
a 15-person family practice group on which the hospital depended heavily for
admissions.

A significant outcome from the retreat was the decision that the success of
the local health care system would ultimately depend on the ability of River
Valley Community Hospital and the Enterprise Medical Group to affiliate with
a larger urban health care system. Such an affiliation would provide access to
larger managed care plans and help secure the futures of both the group and
the hospital. It was considered essential that the group practice and the hospital work closely with one another on this matter.

The hospital and Enterprise developed a plan to interview jointly several
major health care systems in the greater metropolitan area and to evaluate those
systems according to carefully determined criteria. Soon after the retreat, a planning committee of hospital and Enterprise representatives met to explore further
the type of linkage that would be optimal. One approach was for the hospital
and the medical group to develop a joint organization structured as a physician hospital organization. However, Dr. Baker quickly rejected this approach.
She emphasized that her group was looking for an infusion of capital not an
opportunity to invest in a joint venture. Enterprise wanted to sell to the best
bidder. Mr. Young pondered this new event and then concluded that, even if
the hospital could provide the capital, it was not in a position to provide the
long-term salary guarantees requested by the group.

Shortly afterward, Mr. Young received a phone call from Jo Baker, who
conveyed the news that Enterprise's executive committee had decided to

negotiate with interested parties separately from the hospital because of "the sensitivity of the financial issues involved" A quick meeting of the hospital board was called, and tempers began to flare as this news surfaced. Several board members felt betrayed by Enterprise. According to the board chair, Dr. Baker and her colleagues were abandoning the community.

As soon as word was out that Enterprise was for sale, a considerable number of suitors presented themselves, including single-specialty networks, multispecialty networks, and area hospitals. Over about a six-month period, Enterprise narrowed the field and ultimately selected a large urban-based integrated health care system as its choice for a new partner.

As negotiations concluded, Earl Young was somewhat reassured when Jo Baker approached him for input. Dr. Baker wanted to know what special conditions the hospital might like to have added to the agreement that might help protect the hospital, which Dr. Baker pointed out was still very important to the group. One condition from the hospital was that the Enterprise Medical Group needed to understand that the hospital must keep its options open and could not support any exclusive arrangement. The board, in fact, had just directed Mr. Young to seek actively an open dialogue with other health care systems to encourage the presence of other providers in the community. Mr. Young took the week off and contemplated what he should do. He seemed to be caught in a difficult situation. How could he mend relationships with the Enterprise Medical Group, whose admissions to the hospital were crucial, while beginning active recruitment of other providers who would compete with Dr. Baker and her colleagues in the group practice?

Questions for Discussion

1. What factors should be included in developing the criteria for an arrangement between a community health care delivery system and urban health care centers?

2. What are some of the reasons for the Enterprise Medical Group's decision to negotiate separately?

3. What strategies could Earl Young have tried to keep negotiations on track?

4. If you were Earl Young, what would you do now?

CASE 5

Evaluating Emerging Physician-Organization Integration Arrangements

by Howard Zuckerman, Paul R. Torrens,
Diana W. Hilberman, and Ronald M. Andersen

Tree-lined streets, blue skies, band concerts in the park, pollution-
free lakes and streams, and a golf course in almost every town — in
short, northern Iowa is the kind of place where people want to live.
The lifestyle is far removed from the cost, the crime, and the crowds
of larger cities. Warm, friendly, hardworking people will welcome
you with open arms to their communities and their homes.

"Family Care Network"
North Iowa Mercy Health Center

Since 1987, an interesting example of hospital-physician integration has been
gradually evolving in the area around Mason City, Iowa. Begun without great
fanfare, the effort now includes a regional primary care network serving a geographic area with 200,000 people; a regional hospital management and support
system that assists in the operation of small rural hospitals in the region; a
large multispecialty group that is gradually bringing together most of the medical specialists in the region; and a 378-bed regional hospital center formed from
a merger of two previously independent hospitals. Begun in response to expressed community need, this integration has gone forward in a relatively
unforced fashion and has been accompanied by minimal rancor and disagree-
ment between the hospitals and physicians, given the significant nature of the
changes. As such, it provides an important model for consideration by other
rural areas of the United States planning for their future health care systems.

The focus of this case is the development of the Mercy Family Care Network (MFCN) and St. Joseph Mercy Hospital. This case will review the environments within which this network evolved and consider the factors leading to its development, its structure and function, the barriers and facilitators encountered, lessons learned, and implications for the future. Several related initiatives that influenced MFCN will also be examined.

External Environment

Mason City, Iowa is a city of approximately 30,000 set in a lovely agricultural region of northern Iowa near the border with Minnesota. It is the regional center for a 13-county area in which approximately 200,000 people live, and has had a relatively stable population and economy for years. Its distance from other larger cities makes it isolated in some ways, but also makes it more self-sufficient and self-contained. There is a considerable degree of local cohesion, a sense of identity and pride among Iowans in general and in the northern Iowa-Mason City area in particular.

Mason City has served as the regional center for health care for many years. In 1916, the Sisters of Mercy (Detroit Province) established St. Joseph Mercy Hospital in Mason City. In 1978, a small group of medical specialists helped establish a new hospital, the North Iowa Medical Center. Until recently, these two hospitals provided most of the area's primary and secondary care, with more elaborate tertiary care cases sent to Iowa City (or to the Mayo Clinic in Rochester, Minnesota). As will be discussed later, these two hospitals merged in 1993 to form the North Iowa Mercy Health Center (NIMHC).

A well-respected institution, St. Joseph Mercy Hospital has been the key hospital in Mason City, valued by the people of the area as an important part of their community. Although a part of the Mercy Health System, the hospital is viewed by the community as a local institution. General feeling among those interviewed is that the board of trustees of the hospital and its management make decisions based on the needs of the north Iowa community and that the larger system does not interfere in those decisions. The administrative staff at the hospital has been generally stable, with minimal personnel turnover. The CEO has long tenure at the institution, has a good understanding of the people and the medical community in northern Iowa, and is widely respected for his view of the hospital as a broad community health influence in the area.

The supply of physicians in Mason City and the surrounding areas has been generally adequate, in contrast to many other areas of the country in two important respects. There has not been an overabundance of specialists in the community, and specialists there cover a broad range of their individual specialties and have not narrowed their work to subspecialty areas of practice, as often seen in urban areas. However, primary care physicians have been in short supply and the region is considered a rural physician shortage area.

In contrast with many areas, there has not been a great deal of medical competition in Mason City and the surrounding area. Managed care, health maintenance organizations, and other forms of large group purchasing of care have had virtually no penetration yet. Relatively little aggregation of physicians into large groups occurred until recently. The only sense of outside pressure comes from the existence of the Mayo Clinic, about two hours' drive to the north. Indications in the last few years are that the Mayo Clinic may seek to expand its referral network south into the northern Iowa area; to date, such efforts have been limited.

Internal Environment

The organizational culture largely reflects the local community. As is often said, "people live in Mason City because they choose to." Physician recruitment focuses on the upper Midwest to attract individuals who are likely to be homogeneous in the community. Such terms as "homogeneity," "local commitment," and "home-grown" reflect such sentiment. As a result, community and organizational members seem able to communicate with and understand each other well.

In general, relations between the physicians and the hospital in Mason City have been good. Physicians in the immediate community tended to maintain medical staff membership at both of the city's hospitals before their merger, although most physicians concentrated their admissions at one or the other institution. During the 1960s, there was a perception among some specialists that St. Joseph Mercy Hospital was not at the "cutting edge," that it responded too slowly to the environment and did not keep up with important technological advances. This dissatisfaction split the medical community, leading a number of specialists to form the North Iowa Medical Center in 1978. After that time, however, the relationships between both hospitals and their respective medical staffs were largely cooperative in nature. It is noteworthy that one of the frequent comments made about the CEO at St. Joseph Mercy Hospital was that he tried to be sensitive to the needs and the concerns of the physicians on the hospital's medical staff. "The CEO is always welcome in the physicians' lunchroom," commented one physician.

In recent years, St. Joseph Mercy Hospital and its successor organization, the North Iowa Mercy Health Center, have expanded the range of specialty care in Mason City, adding a cardiac surgeon and a supporting cardiology team, a neurosurgeon, and a radiation oncologist. These additions have not only strengthened the organization but have also elevated the level of intensity of medical practice in Mason City.

Historically, the local medical culture has been dominated by specialists who cultivated their referral networks in part through extensive involvement in community social activities. One physician fondly remembers all the ice cream socials he attended. Until recently, the predominant mode of medical practice in Mason City and the surrounding area has been solo or small-group, fee-for-service medical practice, with only one medium-sized group practice and virtually no HMO or managed care practice. Physicians are generally younger than the national average. Physicians do not seem to have overwhelming competitive pressures from other physicians or medical plans; competition is not a major force shaping either medical practice or hospital-physician relations at this time, and physicians are thriving economically. Although Mason City is somewhat removed from other major medical centers (and from Iowa City, where the state university's medical school is located), physicians clearly are conversant with the current developments in medical science and in health care delivery and financing, and have access to and obvious interest in training and exposure outside their geographic area.

There is a long history of effective physician leadership in the community. Two Mason City physicians have served as president of the Iowa Medical Society, and several members of the medical staff have served on the governing boards of the hospital and Mercy Health Services. Importantly, the hospital has had a physician executive as a member of the top management team for years.

The management style or culture at the hospital includes a sense of commitment to the entire 13-county area, of being rooted in the northern Iowa landscape, and of community service. The managerial focus views the various physician-hospital interactions as a critical determinant for the future of the institution. Management also appreciates the importance of physicians to the community and to the hospital. This leads to another important characteristic, an institutional desire to work with the medical staff to build a regional health care system. Finally, the management team feels it is "moving ahead" and "getting things done" for the hospital, creating an atmosphere at NIMHC that suggests change, advancement, progress, and a willingness to innovate and take risk. The management style has been characterized as interactive, consensus-driven, visionary, and empowering. These characteristics will serve well as NIMHC integrates the facility, staff, and programs of the newly consolidated organizations, participates in the merger of the two local multispecialty medical groups — the Mason City Clinic and Park Clinic — and guides the growth of the Mercy Family Care Network, described below.

Development of the Mercy Family Care Network

The Mercy Family Care Network (MFCN) is an integrated network of primary care physicians and the hospital. Initial goals of the network were to help the local communities retain their primary care doctors and, in so doing, enhance the future of these small rural communities. The local rural communities were experiencing a loss of younger physicians who sought a less stressful lifestyle than the 24-hour community coverage they were providing while in solo practice. Joining together in the network would enable them to share coverage, to relieve themselves of many of the administrative burdens of practice, and to ensure a stable income. For the hospital, the network helped formalize relationships with the surrounding rural areas, bring younger physicians into the community, and provide a source of referrals to the hospital and its specialist physicians.

In 1986–87, several family practice physicians in Clear Lake, Iowa became interested in a practice management relationship with the hospital. In response to this interest, the first hospital-physician contract was drafted, leading to hospital ownership and management of the practice, as requested by the physicians. Initial negotiations between the family practice groups and the hospital occurred at the same time that Park Clinic, a local multispecialty medical group, also was attempting to purchase family practices. Thus spurred by the recognition that referrals were flowing to the former North Iowa Medical Center, St. Joseph Mercy Hospital pursued contracting with family practice groups.

Over the next several years, other physicians and physician groups negotiated employment agreements with the St. Joseph Mercy Hospital, each arrangement being somewhat distinctive. The hospital offered physicians a choice among several options, ranging from administrative support, to risk sharing, to full employment. Early participants most often selected the employment option. While being thus linked to the hospital, the physicians had no direct relationship to each other. Recognizing that a more systematic approach was needed, the hospital management invited all physician participants to a retreat in Minneapolis in the fall of 1989. This retreat, and those that would follow regularly, led to a strategic planning process that has guided development of the network.

Several key conclusions have resulted from these retreats, guided by the principles of commitment to a regional system, clinical control by physicians, and shared coverage among participating members. First, the participating primary care physicians began to think of themselves as a single, functioning group practice, closely affiliated with the hospital. The physicians no longer considered themselves as separate, individual practices, but rather viewed themselves as part of a larger whole. The hospital, in turn, moved away from a position of maintaining a series of separate, individual relationships with several practices. Rather, it came to see its role as organizing and coordinating the development of an integrated network of primary care physicians. An important element of the evolution of the network was the role of the St. Joseph CEO who, from 1990 through 1992, met regularly with a representative from each integrated practice. Building on the trust and confidence he had with the physicians, his understanding of the communities, and his skills and knowledge displayed throughout the developmental process, the CEO proved pivotal in the evolution of the network.

Second, an organizational structure emerged that called for the development of regions within the network, each with equal representation, to provide a basis for future collaboration. Currently, there are five such regions, four outside and one within Mason City. By 1992, the formal structure was solidified and bylaws were adopted. Uniform fee schedules and standardized records and procedures were developed and implemented. It was agreed that not only the hospital, but the affiliated physicians' offices also, would subscribe to the standards of the Joint Commission on Accreditation of Healthcare Organizations (JCAHO). Currently, some 60 primary care physicians in Mason City and its 13-county surrounding area participate in MFCN. While the physicians practice in their own communities, the network manages the administrative operations of their practices.

The MFCN is a self-governing unit, treated as a board committee at the hospital. It is dominated by physicians and is responsible for the operational and clinical business of the network, including the range of services, office hours, quality of care, compensation, and physician recruitment. Recently, the governing council has been reorganized to include the five regional representatives, the CEO, the director of the family practice residency program, and the medical director of MFCN. The executive committee includes eight voting members, and the administrative director of MFCN and a physician extender representative serve as nonvoting members. The linkage with the family practice residency program is worth noting. The residency program offers practicing physicians the opportunity to participate in teaching, while providing them with support and coverage within their practices. The program also has proven to be a useful mechanism for physician recruitment.

Concurrent Events

To understand more fully the development and implications of the MFCN, one must understand several initiatives which, while not necessarily directly linked to the network, nevertheless influenced the general atmosphere in the hospital and medical practice in the area. These developments were in large part motivated by a desire to strengthen and improve regional health care and ensure the long-term viability of both the hospital and the physicians. The initiatives included the development of a system for the support of small rural hospitals, development of Centers of Excellence, the merger of St. Joseph Mercy Hospital with the North Iowa Medical Center, and the consolidation of local specialists.

Rural Community Hospital Management

St. Joseph Mercy Hospital has managed under contract a number of small rural hospitals since the middle 1970s. Initially, a small neighboring community hospital in financial distress and at risk of losing its local physicians asked St. Joseph Mercy Hospital to help with its management. Responding to the request, St. Joseph arranged to take complete responsibility for the management and operation of the rural hospital. A pleased community spread the word that St. Joseph Mercy Hospital was shouldering this added involvement in the surrounding counties and, within a few months, a second small community hospital asked for and received assistance and support, although in a slightly different form of organization. By the early 1980s, five hospitals were under contract management with St. Joseph Mercy Hospital.

As each rural hospital situation arose, St. Joseph Mercy Hospital developed administrative solutions tailored to the community's needs. From the beginning, St. Joseph's intent was to serve the needs of the rural communities by supporting the continuation and stabilization of satisfactory health care. St. Joseph did not seek to exploit hospitals that were on hard times, but rather moved carefully so as to be perceived as a good partner. Today, the hospital holds over 150 individual service contracts, as well as management agreements with nine hospitals and 13 clinics. Each managed hospital maintains its own governing board while St. Joseph provides top management, group purchasing discounts, and clinical and support services. The administrator of each managed hospital is a vice president of the NIMHC, thus more fully integrating each of the individual institutions. An important recent advance has linked MFCN physicians to the physician-hospital organizations forming in the managed hospitals outside Mason City.

Centers of Excellence

Another key development was the creation of several tertiary Centers of Excellence. In the early to middle 1980s, much of the tertiary-level care was referred out of the area. To retard the outflow, the hospital sought to upgrade services and develop Centers of Excellence. The hospital recruited several tertiary care specialists in cardiac surgery and cardiology, neurosurgery, and radiation oncology who either wanted to move to Mason City or were looking for new opportunities. In relatively short order, these physicians became the central focus of efforts for special treatment centers in heart disease, neurological problems, and cancer. These centers have been functioning effectively since 1988. In addition, a relationship was formalized with the University of Iowa and, as a result, the cardiac surgeon replicated the Heart Center at Iowa City. This included the cross-training and exchange of heart teams, and the recruitment of a neurosurgeon from the university.

The arrival of these specialists and the development of the Centers of Excellence signaled to Mason City and the surrounding area that the hospital was on the move in important ways. The hospital would come to think in terms of a broader service area, acknowledging that these new specialists would require a more extensive referral base. The changes also signaled a new level of organizational maturity, demonstrating the willingness of the organization to invest its resources to bring new talent and technology to the area.

The creation of the Centers of Excellence reinforced the need for a widespread and well-organized primary care network, as these centers would need a strong, consistent, and reliable referral source of patients. While the MFCN was not developed primarily to bring patients to the centers, it is evident that the network would be a critical component adding significant value through referrals.

Consolidation of Specialists

Historically, specialists in Mason City were organized into solo practice, relatively small groups, or the larger Park Clinic, a multispecialty group operating in Mason City for over 50 years. By 1987, Park Clinic began to include some pediatricians and family practitioners, with the purchase of a primary care practice in Hampton. After being instrumental in developing the former North Iowa Medical Center, Park Clinic began to expand beyond Mason City by purchasing primary care practices in Forrest City, Buffalo Center, and Alison. This led to a noticeable shift in patient flow from St. Joseph Mercy Hospital to the competing North Iowa Medical Center and its affiliated physicians. At issue was how St. Joseph would respond as a number of specialists organized themselves into a group drawing on a rural primary care referral source and with a close association with the other hospital in Mason City.

To counter this outflow of patients, a group of specialists associated with St. Joseph Mercy helped organize the United Hospital Associates, comprising specialists, family practitioners, and the hospital, in order to purchase a competing family practice in Hampton. After this acquisition proved financially unsuccessful, the specialists began the process of creation of what later became the Mason City Clinic. Still convinced of the importance of "getting into the primary care business," the specialists convinced the hospital to commit the financial resources necessary to implement such a strategy. Several respondents suggested that this was, in fact, the seed that ultimately led to the creation of the MFCN.

St. Joseph Mercy Hospital encouraged the creation of a second multispecialty medical group to be closely affiliated with the hospital, in competition with Park Clinic which was affiliated with the North Iowa Medical Center. A number of local specialists, concerned about the future of solo or small-group specialty practice, also favored formation of another multispecialty group. St. Joseph provided these physicians with access to group practice consultants, surveyed land areas near the hospital, selected a site on which to house such a group, and proposed mechanisms by which to integrate the developing MFCN with the multispecialty group. Specialists wanted to affiliate with the hospital that was developing a network that would ultimately influence, if not directly control, much of the specialty care referrals from primary care physicians in the surrounding counties. Formation of the Mason City Clinic adjacent to St. Joseph Mercy Hospital put a majority of the specialists in Mason City in close physical proximity to and solidified the relationship with the hospital. The multispecialty group and the developing primary care network became more closely allied, ensuring the specialists a steady flow of patients from the network.

In early 1993, some physicians from Park Clinic began discussions with St. Joseph Mercy Hospital regarding an affiliation, suggesting they might leave Park Clinic to become members of the MFCN. When the Mason City Clinic leadership was informed about the discussions between St. Joseph and Park

Clinic, they requested that the hospital discontinue its negotiations to allow the Mason City Clinic and Park Clinic to explore alternatives between the two physician groups. Because hospital leaders had encouraged and supported the Mason City Clinic and did not wish to damage carefully nurtured relationships, the hospital withdrew from discussions with the Park Clinic physicians and encouraged them to talk directly with the Mason City Clinic physicians. Reluctantly, Park Clinic began merger discussions with the Mason City Clinic. At about the same time, Park Clinic physicians found that the North Iowa Medical Center was in a difficult financial condition and might have to consider merger or consolidation with St. Joseph Mercy Hospital. In such a circumstance, the Park Clinic physicians would lose their principal hospital and would face problems regarding a primary care network "outside" of the developing MFCN. Merger discussions, while sometimes difficult, were consummated in January 1994. Most of the Park Clinic specialists joined with the Mason City Clinic, with some of the family practitioners and pediatricians joining MFCN.

These developments with the specialists in Mason City had important implications for MFCN. Since MFCN was a part of St. Joseph Mercy Hospital, the hospital now was able to negotiate with virtually all the specialists through the consolidated group from a position of strength and advantage due to its potential to direct referrals. MFCN physicians' commitment was strengthened, and it became increasingly clear that the network was of central importance to the hospital, to referral patterns, and to the collective capability to develop an organized system of care in the Mason City area.

Consolidation of St. Joseph Mercy Hospital and the North Iowa Medical Center

For many years, St. Joseph Mercy Hospital had been the premiere hospital in Mason City. As noted earlier, physician dissatisfaction arose concerning the hospital's ability to maintain a high level of technology. A group of specialists was instrumental in building a new not-for-profit community hospital, the North Iowa Medical Center, the medical staff of which included many of the same physicians who also had privileges at St. Joseph. The new hospital was locally managed until about the middle 1980s, when it contracted with HealthOne, a multihospital system based in Minneapolis. In the late 1980s, the initiatives begun by St. Joseph proved to be highly problematic for the North Iowa Medical Center. In implementing its policy to establish Centers of Excellence, and successfully recruiting a new array of specialists, St. Joseph exceeded the North Iowa Medical Center in the range and depth of its technical capacities. Through management support for rural hospitals and the affiliation with primary care doctors, MFCN, St. Joseph developed and strengthened its base of support and patient referrals from the surrounding regional areas. Finally, support and encouragement of the formation of a large multispecialty group practice, located directly adjacent to the hospital, solidified St. Joseph's standing with the specialists. It became increasingly clear that the community could not support two hospitals and, as the North Iowa Medical Center continued to struggle financially, sentiment for affiliation grew. Discussions eventually led to a consolidation agreement, resulting in the formation of a single operating entity, the NIMH Center. The physical plant of the North Iowa Medical Center would continue to provide outpatient services, long-term care, and other nonacute inpatient services, with acute care services offered at St. Joseph Mercy.

This new consolidated entity would serve to reinforce the directions, initiatives, and purposes of the Centers of Excellence, MFCN, and the multispecialty group practice. MFCN would now play an even more important role as the major source of referrals to the consolidated hospitals and multispecialty physician group. The merger enhanced the strength of the NIMHC in negotiating with primary care doctors from the surrounding areas. Absent unnecessary duplication between two inpatient facilities, the new entity would be stronger financially and would be better able to support MFCN.

Barriers and Facilitators

The development of the Mercy Family Care Network encountered relatively few barriers along the way. Initially, primary care physicians were somewhat reluctant to cede control of their medical practices. Specialists were concerned about the leverage that would accrue to the primary care physicians affiliated with the major hospital and pivotal in the referral network. At the outset, the hospital was inexperienced in managing medical practices. In retrospect, there might have been greater initiative in recruiting primary care physicians and in investing adequate capital resources to build the network.

On the other hand, a number of factors appear to have facilitated network development.

Concern for Community Needs

A key enabling factor was a strong common purpose among all participants to strengthen the health care available to the people of Mason City and the 13-county surrounding area. Those involved realized that community health services would be seriously compromised by the loss of the local hospitals and primary care physicians. Further, without these small, rural hospitals and primary care physicians, the specialists and hospitals in Mason City would suffer as well.

High Level of Trust and Mutual Respect

Following the sense of commitment to the community was an environment of mutual trust and respect by and for the institutions and individuals involved. As a result of NIMHC's long service, the community held it in esteem, and in turn, the institution was clearly linked to the community. Relations between the institution and the physician community, with the exception of a period in the middle 1970s, were seen as positive and constructive.

Homogeneity of Population

The homogeneity of the population was viewed as another factor facilitating the development of the network. Physicians and managers, and their spouses, tended to be drawn from the geographic region. People often locate in Mason City by choice, not by chance, sharing common values, principles, and commitment.

Skilled, Knowledgeable Leadership

In addition, the CEO of the hospital is well known and well respected by the professional community for his technical and managerial competence, his commitment to the geographic area, his general sense of fairness and openness, and his understanding and skill in moving forward the evolution of the network. While disagreements occurred over specific issues, ultimate goals and commitment to physician-organization collaboration were rarely in question. Several physicians with significant leadership abilities and abundant technical knowledge emerged to foster and gain support for the integration effort. These physicians understood the nature of the changes forthcoming in health care, the implications for their region and state, and the advantages of cooperative physician-organization arrangements. The parent system, Mercy Health Services, encouraged and supported the continuing development of physician leadership. The necessity of both managerial and physician leadership to build integrated systems of care is underscored in this case.

Sense of Local Control over Events

The northern Iowa area around Mason City is somewhat isolated and self-contained. Relatively few outside intrusions affected or had significant influence on the development around Mason City. In developing MFCN, participants operated with the understanding that, in large part, they were settling their own fate and helping decide the future of their community. Mercy Health Services, the parent corporation, encouraged this local focus and community sense of ownership in network development.

Natural Evolution of Events

The evolution of events and stages of development are viewed as natural and unforced. St. Joseph Mercy Hospital responded first to the needs of the small rural hospitals and then to the requests from rural primary care physicians for assistance. These efforts subsequently led to a more formalized and expanded primary care network and to further development of the multispecialty group. At several points, when circumstances were viewed as not yet "right," developments were delayed, diverted, or otherwise put aside until the timing was more appropriate. As one key player noted, "events seemed to move along naturally at their own speed, and not according to any one person's game plan."

Market Conditions for Physicians and Hospitals

Finally, these events have taken place in a health care marketplace that has very little managed care or HMO presence. Physicians' incomes were not yet threatened by the immediacy of managed care, nor was the institution facing serious financial danger. Rather, management and physician leaders had a clear understanding of the dynamics of the health care market in the United States, and recognized that similar changes eventually would come to northern Iowa. Thus, the motivating forces were proactive and anticipatory, focusing on long-term concern for the local communities and seeking to position the institutions and physicians for a changing environment.

Challenges for the Future

While much has been accomplished through the events described in and around Mason City, important issues and challenges remain for the institution, physicians, and the community.

Perhaps the overriding issue is how to link together more fully the already established building blocks of an integrated health care system, that is, the primary care network, the multispecialty medical group, and the hospitals. Such a system would be characterized by sharing of risk, responsibility, power, and control across the various organizational and professional groups. Incentives and services will need to be aligned between the consolidated hospitals, between the organization and the physicians, between the primary care and specialist physicians, and within the physician groups. The major challenge, as described by one respondent, is to "connect the dots."

A related issue is the integration of financing and insurance. Although the bases for vertical and horizontal integration of delivery of care are in place, a fully integrated community health care system will ultimately include a financing or insurance component, either through direct ownership or through strategic alliances. Directly linked to the first two challenges is the need for development of an information system with the capability to move health records electronically across all components of the integrated system. Such an information system will eventually provide requisite data in such areas as quality, cost, utilization, practice patterns, clinical outcomes, system performance, and health status. In turn, there arise several financial issues including questions of adequate capital to meet the technological needs of the system and sufficient cash as more primary care physicians move toward salaried arrangements.

The North Iowa Mercy Health Center will also have other issues to address, such as further implementation of continuous quality improvement, evolving roles of governance, the need to retain a system perspective so as not to suboptimize in decision making and resource allocation, facing potential competition at the periphery of its service area, determining how the performance of integrated systems will be defined and measured, and maintaining the collegial organizational and professional culture that has served it so well in developing the system to this point. While these issues and challenges are not trivial, NIMHC has sought to bring together physicians and organizations to build the foundation for a community health care system responsive to the needs of the people it serves.

Questions for Discussion

1. Barriers to the development of the North Iowa Mercy Health Center were seen as relatively modest, largely as a result of environmental and organizational conditions. What would you expect to be the barriers to system development under different conditions?

2. How can managers influence organizational and professional cultures to facilitate the implementation of integrated systems?

3. What approaches might one use to address the future issues facing this system?

4. How are we to define and measure the performance of integrated delivery systems?

Decision Making and Leadership

The Hospital and the Group
Differing Management Styles
at Holy Medical Center

by Nancy M. Friedrich

Holy Medical Center is the oldest hospital in a metropolitan area of two million people. It is located in an upper-income, residential neighborhood. There is an oversupply of both hospital beds and specialty physicians in a market rapidly converting from fee-for-service medicine to prepaid capitated contracts. The service area is predominantly senior citizens, with few young families. Holy Medical Center enjoys a comfortable relationship with its long-term medical staff. Hospital board members, administrators, and senior medical leaders have shared years of collegial relations and Catholic hospital values.

Six independent primary care physicians, all with years of private practice experience, were brought together to form the nucleus for a primary care network. Their sponsor, Holy Medical Center, provided a generous line of credit and income guarantee in return for the physicians' leadership efforts to consolidate office locations and to build office systems that would support an additional 20 primary care practitioners. The six senior physicians were expected to take the lead in recruiting new primary care practitioners to be part of their group, titled Holy Doctors Medical Group (HDMG). The hospital's goal was to use the network to win significant contracts with capitated plans.

During the development of this medical service organization (MSO), the hospital was downsizing to accommodate reductions in both length of stay and admissions. In the process, it assigned one of its "surplus" administrators to head up the new medical group. Dwane Hopkins had a solid history of achievements as a member of the hospital team. He was often the first to volunteer for extra duty, from heading up new task forces to organizing the hospital baseball team.

Unfortunately, Mr. Hopkins was never comfortable with physicians. He often clashed over minor procedural and policy issues. While these clashes were frequently the subject of surgeons' lounge talk, they never came to the attention of the chief operating officer (COO) of the hospital. As far as the COO was concerned, Mr. Hopkins's record of cooperation and team contribution made him the perfect candidate to adjust hospital systems to support the group.

Since the signing of the MSO, the physicians had no feedback on the financial status of their practice. When the busiest physician asked, Mr. Hopkins would say, "I haven't been able to get the finance department to produce any reports yet." When the group's medical director asked Sister Margaret, president and chief executive of the medical center, she said, "Oh, don't worry; we're in this for the long haul."

Eight months after the formation of HDMG, the COO realized the new medical group had made no progress on consolidation or physician recruitment. In fact, the COO realized the HDMG physicians hardly knew Mr. Hopkins, who remained entirely outside of the daily operating routine of the six physicians in their three separate offices. Mr. Hopkins was asked to resign. The medical center advertised for and hired a group practice manager with considerable experience in group practice management and prepaid plan management.

Lucy Simmons arrived on the job with years of practical experience in unraveling doctor financial and productivity disasters. Her first job was to get the medical center finance department to produce financial statements for the Holy Doctors Medical Group. Six weeks after Ms. Simmons began her new job, she received an eight-month budget and two balance sheets: one for HDMG (patient revenue and physician salaries and benefits) and one for the holding company (all other practice expenses such as employee salaries and benefits, rent, and office and medical supplies). Separately or combined, however, the balance sheets did little to illuminate the group's financial performance for the new administrator. Nor was the eight-month budget-to-actual report very meaningful. The HDMG budget had been built for rapid expansion. Both budgeted revenues and budgeted expenses were much higher than actual. And when Ms. Simmons went back to the finance department to request data on billing and accounts receivable, she was put off with a variety of excuses.

Ms. Simmons' next level of analysis included asking for productivity data such as clinic and hospital visits, by physician. When she could not get that information out of the financial records, she went to the office staff who booked the appointments. After several hours of tallying visits from the appointment book and looking up inpatient visits from charts, Ms. Simmons was able to construct the matrix shown in Table 1.

She shared the matrix with each physician individually. She was surprised that they all accepted the data with a shrug and no argument. The medical director of the group, who was also well respected as chief of medicine at Holy Medical Center, mused that some of his medical center responsibilities kept him from scheduling clinic time two afternoons a week. Furthermore, when the ink was dry on the MSO contract, he had dropped off another afternoon of practice in the clinic to play golf as, after two years of meeting two and three

Table 1. Production Report, Holy Doctors Medical Group
January 1 through August 31

Physician	Clinic Half-Days per Week	Fee-for-Service Encounters	+ Hospital Encounters	+ Managed Care Encounters	= 8-Month Total Encounters	12-Month Total Encounters
#1	4.5	936	173	172	1,281	1,922
#2	4.5	1,107	44	205	1,356	2,034
#3	4.0	1,052	507	194	1,753	2,630
#4	5.0	1,797	50	85	1,932	2,898
#5	8.5	1,283	73	109	1,465	2,198
#6	8.5	719	50	153	922	1,383
TOTAL		6,894	897	918	8,709	13,065

Medical Group Management Association Mean Family Practice Visits: 5,613
Medical Group Management Association Mean Internal Medicine Visits: 4,740
HDMG Mean Visits: 13,065/6 = 2,178

nights a week with attorneys and consultants to develop the MSO, he felt justified in taking a "breather."

After eight weeks on the job, Ms. Simmons and the finance department had pulled together enough financial data to know the following: in its first eight months, the group had lost $91,400. If trends continued, the loss would be $137,100 by year end.

In addition, Ms. Simmons had identified personality problems with one of the members of the group. He was threatened by talks to recruit new physicians because his own practice was not full. Every time a new physician showed interest in joining the group, Dr. Slow quietly sabotaged the recruitment efforts.

Questions for Discussion

1. Why did Dwane Hopkins fail as a clinic manager?
2. Was the hospital CEO too harsh in discharging Mr. Hopkins?
3. Why couldn't the hospital's finance department produce timely reports for the clinic?
4. What could have been done to solve the productivity problem?
5. What are some of the key factors that should be included in a contract or arrangement between a hospital and an acquired group practice?

CASE 7

Organization Conflict
Strong Department Heads versus Central Administration

by Joel Koemptgen

Academically oriented group practices struggle with attaining the proper balance between departmental control and central administrative governance. Medical department leaders at times confuse managing their departmental operations, which is their responsibility, with setting or interpreting policy, which is the appropriate role of the board and administration. Conversely, the board and administration attempt to dictate or interpret operational strategy to departments that do not welcome this perceived interference in their internal affairs.

Prior to 1985, this hospital-based group practice functioned like a typical university-based faculty practice. Strong department heads exhibited significant independence, often negotiating the terms of their relationship to the hospital and affiliated university as well as entering into independent contracts with outside organizations and third party providers.

In 1984, a physician president was recruited from outside of the group to create a strong group-practice model. He survived less than two years. Department heads who had long tenure within the organization, some of whom were on the board but most of whom were not, led a palace revolt that resulted in the firing of the president. Within the next year, other physician leaders who had been supportive of the president found themselves in disfavor, and those of them who were board members were eventually removed from the board. During this same period, a number of key administrative people resigned or were encouraged to do so.

In 1987 a "caretaker" was appointed interim president of the physician group. He was a longtime member who had little administrative experience, but who appeared to be acceptable to most factions within the organization.

Over the next year, he assembled an experienced administrative team and enthusiastically set out to build a solid group-practice organization.

This physician organization is a nonprofit, 180-physician, hospital-affiliated group practice with strong ties to a major university. The physician practice, which is affiliated and physically connected with a 455-bed teaching hospital, is one of three subsidiary organizations under a common, nonoperational parent. The nonprofit parent board receives and ratifies the budgets of the subsidiaries, approves major initiatives such as strategic planning, and acts as arbiter if disputes cannot be settled at the subsidiary board level.

The group practice includes all major medical and surgical specialties. There is also a significant primary care representation that includes residency programs in internal medicine, pediatrics, and family medicine.

The group practice is governed by a board of directors and a central administrative staff. (Please see organizational chart, Figure 1.) It is commonly acknowledged, however, that a "shadow government" exists among the medical department heads. Even though a majority of the 11-member board is composed of department chairs, they rarely take actions that would be contrary to any of the departments' wishes.

The department chairs, or their equivalent for outside contract departments, report to both the president of the clinic and the president of the medical center. The nature of their joint appointments, along with their status as clinical faculty at the affiliated university, contribute to the perception that the department chairs lack loyalty to the clinic board and administration. Additionally, many of the larger departments have their own professional administrative staffs, who report directly to the chair of the department but have no reporting relationship to the central clinic administration.

The central administrative staff report directly through the administrative chain of command, but are also expected to respond directly to the requests of the department heads, even if there are conflicts in perceived goals or strategies. The inconsistency in reporting arrangements between the medical and administrative leaders causes stress within the organization.

With a dual administrative structure also comes some duplication of cost. Within the medical departments, significant amounts of the physician department heads' time are devoted to administration. Given the fact that the department heads are the highest-compensated individuals within their departments, and the fact that they are not generating clinical income as administrators, it is clear that costs of this group practice are higher than in private practice and that, generally, production is somewhat less. Add to this the presence of professional administrative staff as noted above, and administrative overhead in many of the departments becomes significant.

The administrative cost burden to the organization would be more reasonable if a large layer of central administrative staff and other costs were not overlaid on the aforementioned medical department administrative overhead. The costs of central administration, including a nearly full-time physician

Figure 1. Organizational Chart

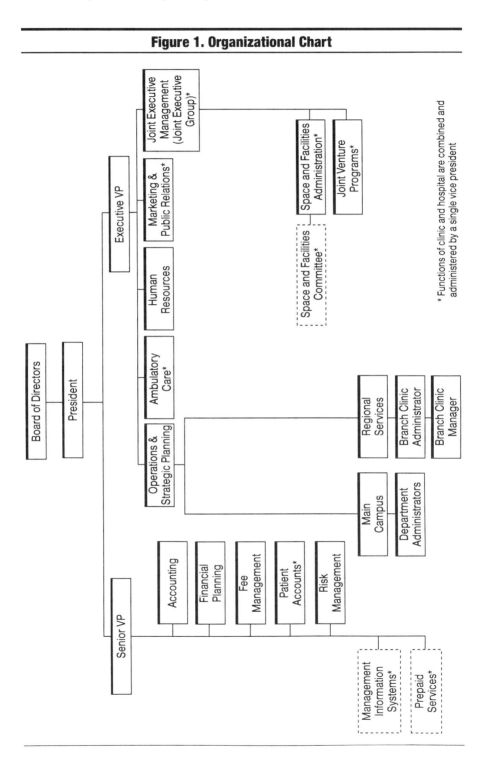

president, approach those of other large groups within the Medical Group Management Association.

The cost structure noted above would be acceptable if reimbursement was sufficient to cover the additional overhead of the dual system. Unfortunately, a majority of clients are eligible for either Medicaid or Medicare, and an additional 10 percent are truly indigent. Since roughly 60 percent of the patient mix is reimbursed at 50 percent or less of fee-for-service charges, the remaining 40 percent of patients must unrealistically make up much of the difference. The only positive offset is a physician services reimbursement agreement with the medical center for teaching and department administrative services. The combination of the low fee-for-service reimbursement and the limited dollars from the physician services agreement contributed to a $1 million operating loss for the clinic in 1989.

In addition to reporting and cost issues, the academic model often labors under conflicting decision-making processes. Often it is unclear whether department heads or central administration should initiate strategies. Questions often arise as to what is appropriately a departmental strategy versus an organizational strategy. And if the two strategies are in conflict, it is not obvious which one takes precedence. Generally, though certainly not exclusively, strategies initiated by the departments tend to be politically motivated, whereas central administrative initiatives tend to be driven by bottom-line considerations.

The dual decision-making system consumes more time than a traditional, vertically administered organization. Task forces, committees, and consensus are the preferred decision-making processes for this academic group practice organization.

Added to this less-than-optimal decision making process is the reality of an inadequate management information system. A poorly automated and understaffed management information department undermines the timeliness and appropriateness of decision making at all levels of the organization.

A number of alternatives were explored for dealing with the problems enumerated above. The three most significant were:

1. Reductions of selected administrative positions
2. Voluntary shifts in operational leadership to either a more centralized or a more decentralized structure
3. A formal governance review, with the anticipated outcome being substantive changes

The chosen course of action was a mix of all three alternatives. The process for seeking change was hastened by two unfortunate events: the sudden death of the president of the clinic and the realization of a $4 million budget shortfall — both of which occurred in early 1990.

Overcoming a $4 million deficit required large cuts in administrative and departmental budgets. A painful process was initiated, with cuts in all areas except physician compensation. The latter area was spared only because the clinic was losing valued physicians at the rate of nearly one in five per year. Cuts were made in central administration in both a planned and an unplanned fashion. Two vice presidents elected to leave rather than participate in what they alleged to be a dismantling of the group-practice structure. A third vice president was removed from his position and made to report to the hospital chief financial officer.

During this period of instability in the central administrative structure, a governance task force was appointed. It was felt by some that this was equivalent to shutting the barn door after the horses had escaped. The charge to the governance task force is included as Exhibit 1.

Exhibit 1. Charge to the Governance Task Force

The Governance Task Force is charged to address the following:

- To evaluate the working relationship of the clinic to its parent organization and to the other subsidiaries

- To review the clinic bylaws, as currently stated, for purposes of determining if it is governing itself in the most appropriate manner (i.e., the roles of the president, board of directors, senior management, and department heads)

- To evaluate the relevance of 1989 board accomplishments related to stated goals and objectives (focus on governance relationships versus operations)

- To explore ways and means of achieving greater participation and support from the clinic physician membership at large toward the attainment of clinic organizational initiatives

- To discern if there is an organizational structure that lends itself to optimal reimbursement by third party payers

- To determine if there are certain departments or functions within the clinic whose financial performance could be enhanced sufficiently to justify the creation of a for-profit subsidiary

- To consider ways and means of enhancing central and departmental administrative functions and responsibilities

- To evaluate the relationship of the clinic to the university and reassess the commitment of the organization to research and education.

As of this writing, the task force has met on three occasions; however, it continues merely to restate problems without identifying meaningful solutions. It is expected that the final report will not be completed for a number of months. In the meantime, the administrative reorganization has already been undertaken. Financial leadership has been given to the medical center in an acknowledgment that the clinic will function more like a federation of departments than like a traditional group practice.

The clinic's governance experiences of the last five years have taught the organization three valuable lessons.

1. Be what you want to be.

2. Combining centralized and decentralized administration is inefficient.

3. Dual governance can foster high staff turnover.

For over 40 years, the physicians have constituted, historically and culturally, a hospital-based, university-affiliated practice. As such, they are more comfortable with a consensus-based, process-oriented governance structure that values the individual department over the central organization. Given that focus, there is often a distrust of centralized decision-making processes.

Experience has also taught the physician leaders that the combination of centralized and decentralized administration works rather poorly — it is inefficient, expensive, and slow to act and often produces ambiguous results. Physicians and department heads assume a we/they attitude toward the central board and administration, which leads to distrust from both perspectives. Finally, many physicians and administrators are confused as to who is ultimately responsible for carrying out the policies of the organization and of the departments. Physician reporting lines are clear — through section chiefs to department heads to the president of the clinic. Unfortunately, these lines are not as clear for administrative personnel; department administrators report to the department heads, and central administrators report to the clinic president, with little coordination of activities between the two.

The third lesson is perhaps the most painful of all — dual governance fosters high staff turnover. Action-oriented leaders, both within the departments and within central administration, become frustrated with the lack of decisive decision making. Turf battles between departments and central administration lead to distrust and bitterness. This distrust between the two administrative entities creates significant difficulty in building the positive corporate culture needed to enhance recruitment and retention. Within the last five years, there has been nearly 100 percent turnover of physician staff, with central administrative staff turnover nearly as high.

In summary, academically oriented physicians and physician leaders are generally not advocates of strong centralized organizational processes. Attempts over a five-year period at integrating departmental and central administrative functions have been considered, by and large, a failure.

Alternative strategies for reducing selected administrative overhead, voluntary shifting of operational leadership to a more centralized or a more decentralized style, and formal governance review were all considered as options in dealing with the stated problem. A combination of the three alternatives has been chosen, with the direction being toward a more decentralized system.

The physician group now accepts its historical and cultural base and no longer considers a strong central governance to be its focus. And since the combination of centralized and decentralized administration is inefficient, costly, and sometimes confusing, it is apparent that a smaller, more focused centralized administration will be the outcome of the present organizational review process.

Questions for Discussion

1. Perform a SWOT (strengths, weaknesses, opportunities, threats) analysis of the administrative and governance problems encountered in this case, and identify the three problems you consider to be the most significant.

2. How would you develop your strategy for resolving these problems?

3. Why do physicians appear at times to oppose centralization of management and decision making?

4. As an executive, what steps can you take to reduce unnecessary friction between physicians who oppose centralization and lay executives or physician executives who are interested in centralizing authority?

5. Review the charge to the Governance Task Force. If you were the executive preparing this charge, would you have drafted it any differently? If so, how and why?

CASE 8

Integrating the Skilled Nursing Unit at Best HMO

by Susan Tuller and Therese M. Martaus

Janet Adams, manager of finance and planning for Best Health Maintenance Organization (BHMO), brought her presentation to the executive administrative group to a close. Dr. Robert Martin, assistant medical director for the HMO, sat glaring across the table. He had just finished an angry speech condemning both the organization's new skilled care facility, Vernon Care Center, and the report she had presented of her staff's evaluation of the facility's performance. His criticisms were not uncommon at this table, around which sat senior administrators from each service delivery area and support function of the organization, including the medical staff director and assistant director, the director of quality of care and service, the director of care and utilization management, the nursing administrator, the coordinator of ancillary services, the hospital service administrator, and the director of home and skilled care services.

Dr. Martin declared that the report had been written without his knowledge or support and did not adequately represent physician views of the facility. He cited several specific concerns, not the least of which were quality of care, cost per patient day, and lack of communication between providers at the facility and their colleagues in the rest of the organization. Ms. Adams responded by offering a list of the physicians who had been contacted for input into the report. The executive vice president, who chaired the meeting, called for recess.

The goal of the report had been: (1) to bring closure to the startup phase of operations for Vernon Care Center by evaluating how well the facility met its original planning goals of providing quality care and assisting in care and utilization (and therefore cost) management for the HMO as a whole, and (2) to provide groundwork for ongoing planning for the facility as an integral part of the organization's continuum of care. Ms. Adams believed that the success of the report would be measured by its credibility and by the level of acceptance it achieved among the different groups and perspectives involved.

However, as had been demonstrated to her throughout the process of preparing this report, perceptions of achievement and performance were often driven by the individual or group perspectives of the disciplines and functions represented at this senior administrative table. In fact, each senior administrator present had a bone to pick with the new facility. BHMO placed a high degree of value on incorporating all available input and perspective, so it had been the job of her staff to sort through the assumptions and individual agendas of this complex organization and synthesize them in their report. Their failure with Dr. Martin was obvious. Janet Adams had two concerns as she left the meeting: first, that she reach Dr. Martin and address his concerns; and second, that she assess the possible effect and credibility of Dr. Martin's response throughout the organization.

The Organization

BHMO is a regional company providing care to approximately 500,000 members in two states. The organization is both insurer and health care provider for its members, providing services in BHMO-owned facilities and clinics for a fixed, prepaid fee. The vast majority of its Medicare members are covered through a Tax Equity and Fiscal Responsibility Act (TEFRA) risk-sharing arrangement.

BHMO operates its own hospitals, medical specialty centers, and primary care medical centers throughout its geographic service area. It also owns and operates several home care agencies, which provide home health and hospice care. Additionally, BHMO contracts with a long-term care service to provide primary care to BHMO members living in residential long-term care settings. As an insurer and medical care provider, the HMO also contracts with area inpatient facilities such as hospitals and skilled nursing facilities for specialty services and postacute skilled care.

Skilled Care at the HMO

As noted above, BHMO members requiring skilled care receive that care in a number of settings. Despite its prepaid, capitated system of financing health care services, and its TEFRA contract, BHMO follows Medicare guidelines in its administration and coverage of care in a skilled nursing facility (SNF). Any skilled nursing care to be covered under Medicare Part A (SNF-A) requires a three-day qualifying stay in an acute care setting, and a daily need for skilled nursing or rehabilitation services as certified by a physician. As BHMO moved to decrease acute care costs, the role of the SNF and the need for easy access to that setting became increasingly important. Original planning documents for BHMO's own skilled care facility showed that the primary reason for opening this facility was ready access to quality, skilled care beds. It was expected that a BHMO-owned SNF would assure timely access to necessary Medicare SNF-A beds.

At the time Vernon Care Center was acquired, the HMO was experiencing difficulty placing patients in skilled nursing facilities in the community. Several reasons for this were identified:

- A limited number of skilled care facilities were Medicare-certified in BHMO's central service area in 1990.

- Higher acuity and earlier hospital discharge had resulted in a significant increase in the intensity of skilled care requirements for members.

- It was especially difficult to place patients with complex wound and skin care, multiple-IV medication management, and complex psychosocial issues.

- Area SNFs accused BHMO of paying too little for patients with higher acuity needs.

- Internal case managers reported delayed admissions to skilled nursing facilities due to "nursing home procedures" and complained of an inability to admit patients on weekends or holidays, or after hours.

Further, access to SNF-A beds was expected to become increasingly problematic in the near future. This was a result of growing BHMO needs for SNF-A beds and of the state's response to an increasing demand for long-term skilled nursing care beds, including both long-term care and SNF-A.

- In 1989, the state health coordination council decreased the number of allowable nursing home beds from 53 per 1,000 population to 45 per 1,000 population.

- BHMO's planning department estimated long-term care bed need (at the 45 per 1,000 rate set by the council) at 1,424 beds in 1991, 1,645 beds in 1995, and 1,817 beds in 2000.

- BHMO estimated its need for Medicare SNF-A beds to be 100 (on average daily) in 2000, approximately double the 1989 demand.

BHMO also recognized the relationship between access to SNF-A beds and utilization management of hospital days and organizational financial performance, and identified several key areas where a BHMO-owned facility might have influence.

- The cost of SNF-A days in the community was expected to increase due to loss of intermediate care beds and increased demand for long-term care and SNF-A beds.

- High hospital census with patients at a nonacute level of care in acute care beds led to: (1) patients being diverted to external hospitals and

(2) higher variable cost per day for patients at a nonacute level of care if they were in a hospital rather than at an SNF-A.

- That same variable cost could be saved for patients awaiting long-term permanent placement if they waited in an SNF-A setting rather than in a hospital.

Vernon Care Center

In 1991, BHMO entered into an agreement to purchase an SNF located in a major urban area, geographically in the heart of the HMO's service area. Working with outside experts, BHMO made modifications to the facility and plant operations in an effort to bring the facility in line with the higher-acuity patients that BHMO expected to admit to the Medicare SNF-A unit.

The facility is designed to provide nursing and rehabilitation services to those patients requiring skilled, nonacute care. As is the case with the HMO's acute inpatient facilities, administrative policy requires that all eligible enrollees receive care at the facility. This is a change from BHMO's traditional practice of admitting patients to a number of non-HMO SNFs and contracting for those services as an insurer. Still, exceptions to this policy are made, based on care needs that cannot be met by the facility or the presence of a spouse or partner in another long-term care facility. The HMO contracts or arranges all other SNF care through other licensed care facilities.

Vernon Care Center opened with high expectations that it would "find its place" in BHMO's continuum of services. After several months, it became apparent that there were extensive gaps in the coordination of care and services for patients served at the facility. Facility staff complained that they did not receive medical information in a timely way; care management monitors in the acute care setting cited limited bed availability at Vernon Care Center as a serious obstacle to their efforts in managing patient acute care appropriately. Stories of consumer complaints resulting from some of these missteps filtered back to providers in other care settings, including medical staff who were unfamiliar with SNF procedures or SNF-A coverage requirements.

Additionally, higher acuity needs than originally anticipated led nursing administration to ask for greater staff support, meaning that the cost per day at the facility was considerably higher than originally projected. Many players in the organization believed that these were "growing pains." As hospital lengths of stay decreased, the number of admissions to the facility increased — at greater patient acuity. The volume of admissions to the facility was more than double what had been anticipated. Vernon Care Center was designed as an SNF to reduce the need to place members in external facilities, where care could not be managed from a medical or utilization standpoint. However, Vernon Care Center was not a traditional SNF although it conformed with Medicare regulatory requirements. Thus, there was ongoing confusion about its role and its capabilities to provide long-term care and the increasingly demanding skilled care that evolved into an intermediate level called "transitional care."

Toward the end of the first year of the facility's operations, tensions in some areas of the BHMO were so high and the staff morale at the facility was so poor, that it was necessary to find some way to communicate organizational attention and awareness of the issues and to identify a plan for addressing them.

At year end, Janet Adams was asked to develop a one-year evaluation of the startup of the quality and care management of the facility, to be presented to senior administration at the quarterly meeting in March.

The Process of Evaluation

BHMO's organizational culture required some type of collective evaluation process in keeping with the high value it placed on inviting all interested parties into a dialogue in policymaking. Knowing this, Janet Adam's first task had been to develop a work plan for the evaluation, which included identifying key players or individuals who would have interest in decision making around the facility. The work plan outlined goals for the facility in the areas of quality and utilization, the scope of the evaluation analysis, and the resources she proposed to use to measure the facility's overall performance. She made sure that the facility managers and administrators, including the Vernon Care Center medical director, Dr. Luke O'Connor, approved the work plan. She also presented it to the organization's oversight group for SNF planning, and to the senior administrative group for their additions and comments. Each of these groups had added questions, concerns, and issues to the evaluation work plan.

By January, the work of evaluation was begun in earnest. Janet Adams and her staff reviewed all available written material regarding the planning for the facility and its performance through the first year of operations, including financial and utilization management reports. Their analysis included a review of patient satisfaction survey results. They also reviewed the results of an employee survey. Those surveyed included physicians whose patients were admitted to Vernon Care Center, hospital discharge planners, and home care staff involved when patients were discharged from the facility.

In addition, Luke O'Connor gave Ms. Adams the names of ten physicians to interview for their specific input. A telephone survey was created for these physicians, to be administered by the planning staff. Despite the fact that Dr. O'Connor had drafted a memo requesting his colleagues to cooperate with these interviews, only four physicians completed the telephone survey. Finally, planning staff pulled a draft report together and reviewed it with those who had contributed, to confirm their input. Dr. Martin was not among those interviewed.

Next Steps

At the end of the meeting with senior administration, Janet Adams was concerned that despite the careful work of her staff in bringing together information and different constituencies from throughout the organization, they had not been successful enough in ferreting out all the serious past concerns and issues to allow the organization to begin planning for the facility's role in the future.

Questions for Discussion

1. Why was Dr. Martin so upset about the evaluation report, and what could have been done differently to preclude the problem?

2. Were there any pieces missing from the evaluation process?

3. What are the functions of program evaluation within an organization?

4. Why did the state health coordinating council decrease the number of available nursing home beds from 53 per 1,000 population to 45 per 1,000 population?

CASE 9

Evolution of Leadership

by Chad L. Peter

As if questing for the Holy Grail, the Shasta Group Practice has been in constant search for the right combination of leadership and governance to set and achieve organizational goals for the entire 32 years of its existence. By the time Janet Smith became administrator, the group had moved through two distinct types of autocratic leadership. It had never developed a strong foundation for democratic governance and leadership, and in Ms. Smith's opinion it was unequipped to do so. Ms. Smith believed that such a form and style would be necessary to meet the challenges ahead, particularly disagreements over the income distribution plan and whether to expand from a multidisciplined primary care group to a true multispecialty group. The Shasta Group needed consistent, effective leadership so that it could develop a corporate philosophy that a large majority of its physicians would back. It also needed well-defined goals and objectives to put that philosophy into practice. Without that type of leadership, she believed the group would continue to founder. Too many physicians would be lost to stronger groups.

The management styles the group has experienced include: (1) the benevolent physician dictator, (2) the power broker lay administrator, and (3) several stages of democratic processes. Now it is developing physician leaders for the executive board.

Benevolent Physician Dictator

At the beginning, the group grew from the vision of a very generous and benevolent physician. This physician trained at the Mayo Clinic and brought back to the community the conviction that the future of medicine was going to be in group practice. He and his brother-in-law, who was also a physician in the community, agreed to form an eight-physician, multidisciplined group practice. To fulfill the administrative duties of this new organization, the physicians hired John Hawley, an accountant who had previously worked with several of them.

Leadership for this new group consisted of a benevolent dictator, Dr. Will Means, who made all the decisions for the lay administrator to implement. Mr. Hawley defined this style of leadership as benevolent dictatorship because "Dr. Will" controlled the group and decision making. He had a generous, humanitarian nature, and he held the respect of all the physicians. It was not uncommon for him to reduce his own salary to help a young physician over rough times. He was also generous with the community, serving on many boards and giving freely of himself to community affairs. Dr. Will was highly respected, and that made his leadership effective.

Strengths
Some of the strengths of this style of leadership were that:

- Decisions were made quickly without time-consuming debate.
- Meetings were relatively infrequent.
- Physicians enjoyed being freed from business concerns so they could concentrate on medicine.
- The group's respect for the leader and his decision-making ability created cohesiveness.
- The decisions typically benefited the majority: "the tail never wagged the dog."

Weaknesses
Weaknesses of the benevolent dictatorship included that:

- Decisions were unilateral, made without input from others.
- Succession planning was poor. Other physicians were not developing leadership skills.
- Ideas, while not discouraged, were not encouraged and nurtured.

Power Broker Lay Administrator

When Dr. Will retired, there was a void in physician leadership. Since none of the physicians had been groomed and developed to assume the leadership, the authority fell by default to John Hawley, the lay administrator. Mr. Hawley had developed his leadership style while serving as the benevolent dictator's first lieutenant, and as a result he became a power broker administrator. Mr. Hawley defined a power broker as a person who exerts strong influence through the individuals or votes he controls. This leadership style developed from the mentoring relationship between Mr. Hawley and Dr. Will.

The power broker style worked at first because the physicians were used to following, and following the administrator's lead was business as usual.

During this period, Mr. Hawley played a powerful role in the group. The physicians had respect for his strong business acumen, but overall this was an era when administration was considered a necessary evil.

Mr. Hawley's style of leadership worked fairly well until new physicians joined the group. New physicians in the 1970s and 1980s wanted more input into business decisions. Mr. Hawley, as a power broker administrator, was deeply entrenched, and many physicians felt that they were working for him rather than the other way around. New physicians became frustrated with the administrator, and also with senior partners. For example, senior partners would agree with the young physicians on what should be done but would avoid confrontation with the administrator. The dominance that Mr. Hawley had over the business affairs was very difficult to dislodge. This controversy between the administration and the physicians affected the effectiveness of the practice.

Strengths
Advantages to the group during this time of power brokering included that:

- The administrator's keen business sense kept the group making forward progress.
- The autocratic style of the administrator gave him the ability to act quickly on decisions.
- The administrator had the freedom to negotiate with sources of outside pressures without checking with a board.
- The administrator provided leadership in a period when physician leadership was underdeveloped.

Weaknesses
On the other hand, because of this style of leadership:

- Physicians were not involved in leadership.
- The junior partners' lack of respect and acceptance for the administrative approach fueled controversy.
- The group began to lose direction and purpose.
- Several young physicians left the group.

Stages of Democratic Development
John Hawley took early retirement, and Janet Smith was hired as the new administrator. Ms. Smith was familiar with the benevolent dictator and power broker styles of management and knew the problems associated with both of them. She recognized the need to move the physicians toward a new, more democratic form of governance and leadership. Her goals were (1) to develop

key physician leaders, and (2) to develop physician ownership of decisions through involvement in making and implementing the decisions.

Executive Board Dominance

The first stage of leadership transition was to develop a strong and active executive board. This board consisted of six physician representatives, one from each clinical area. Weekly meetings were held to discuss, and to make decisions on, all facets of the group practice. Physician interest and involvement grew steadily as the board made decisions previously made by the administrator.

Strengths
This form of leadership had its strengths:

- Physicians on the executive board were involving themselves in decisions.
- A new sense of ownership developed among the board physicians.
- Decisions were made in a timely fashion because the board met weekly.
- Administration developed a more cooperative role with the physicians.

Weaknesses
It also had its share of weaknesses:

- Physicians were not always being represented by the most qualified physician. Seats on the executive board were passed around on a rotation basis.
- While the physicians on the board were involved in the leadership process, the rest of the physicians on the staff had very little involvement. Many were starting to resent the decisions of the board in the same way they had resented decisions of the power broker administrator.
- The executive board made too many small decisions that should have been left up to the administrator. For example, the board spent more time discussing whether the laboratory director should have a $50 beeper than whether to purchase a $50,000 item.
- The administrator was responsible for preparing the entire agenda and carrying out the decisions on a weekly basis. Ms. Smith felt she spent too much time on bureaucracy and paperwork at the expense of more important activities.

Development of a Standing Committee Structure

The second stage of leadership transition was to expand the role of the general staff under the executive board. This addressed the dissatisfaction among physicians who were not on the executive board and felt they were not being given enough influence over decisions. A system of standing committees was formed and charged with overseeing specific areas of the practice, such as personnel. The standing committees were accountable to the executive board. Every physician was assigned to a committee. Each committee met monthly and provided regular reports to the board.

Strengths
Positive aspects of this arrangement were that:

- Physicians were now contributing to the decision-making process of the group.
- The physician members were developing a sense of ownership.
- More physicians had the opportunity to develop leadership skills by serving as committee chairs.

Weaknesses
On the negative side:

- The executive board continued to meet weekly to make decisions that should have been studied by a standing committee first.
- Over time, the physicians began to lose interest in their committees because they simply got tired of meetings.
- Committees were not politically savvy enough to accept that an occasional defeat is a normal part of the process. Whenever the executive board turned down a committee's recommendation, committee members became angry. This contributed to their losing interest in the committee system.
- Paperwork more than doubled for the limited administrative staff, which had to prepare materials for all the committees.
- Because of Ms. Smith's detailed involvement with all committees and the executive board, she was still playing too much of a leadership role in Shasta. While she enjoyed this position, the group needed to develop a key physician leader who would have the respect of his or her colleagues both in medicine and in business.

Task Forces
Eventually, the committee structure was replaced with task forces. The task forces report to the executive board. When the assignment is completed, the task force is dissolved. The physicians respond much better to this solve-the-problem approach.

Strengths
Among the strengths of this approach are that:

- Physicians are able to focus on a specific, narrow problem and find a workable solution. The success rate is high.
- Meetings are called on an as-needed basis. The task forces have eliminated the routine, monthly committee meetings.
- Task force members can be appointed who have specific interest and expertise in the problem being addressed.

Weaknesses
The downside of task forces is that:

- The executive committee is still handling too many problems that could be better studied by a task force.
- Physicians on the general staff are not as participatory as they were with the standing committee structure.
- In naming task forces, there is a tendency to keep choosing the same willing physicians.

Physicians in Management

The Shasta Group Practice is developing physician leaders for the executive board. One key to developing physician leadership is the physician-in-management courses that have become available around the country. Shasta's physician president eventually completed the entire program. This has proved to be a pathway that brings a new level of physicians into management. As administrator, Ms. Smith finds it easier to discuss issues with management-oriented physicians because they have a greater understanding of the business side of medicine. Today the Shasta Group requires that all members of the executive board complete at least two courses in management.

Strengths

The strengths of this policy include that:

- Physician board members now have a better understanding of the management side of medicine.
- Physician leaders are surfacing.
- Physicians and lay administrators are working better as a team.

Weaknesses

The policy also has weaknesses:

- Only board members have taken the courses. Not everyone is willing to support the decisions of the elected leaders and administration when those decisions — however managerially sound — mean unwelcome change for an individual.
- Even physicians who took some management courses have trouble applying what they learned.
- Decisions are still being made in part according to physicians' personal biases rather than business sense.
- When tough decisions are made, the general staff still tends to second guess leadership.

Summary

The Shasta Group Practice has been searching for the proper combination of leadership and management styles to steer the group into the future. The group has been through several styles of autocratic and democratic leadership. What the group found in its quest for this Holy Grail was that the goal is unachievable. People and circumstances change; what worked well yesterday may not succeed tomorrow. Victory is in the quest for perfection.

Questions for Discussion

1. Do you agree with the strategy Janet Smith employed to turn the management and governance practices around? Would you have done anything differently? If so, what?

2. Drawing from your knowledge of organizational behavior, how would you classify the management styles experienced by this group?

3. What are the major reasons for the failure of the standing committee structure? How would you make standing committees more successful if you had been the administrator?

Clinical and Managerial
Quality Improvement

.

CASE 10

A Winning Game Plan for CQI

by Robert Boyle, Jr.

The days of macromanagement in health care are numbered. Medical group administrators can no longer rely on their ability to expand revenues by increasing the client base, adding physicians, or tweaking fees. Instead, the major challenge facing health care management today is to do more with less. Given this challenge, in late 1991, West Coast Clinic began to think about continuous quality improvement (CQI) as an answer. The clinic has over 100 physicians and is located in northern California.

Shortcomings of Existing CQI Programs

To find out what some of the pitfalls in a CQI effort might be, West Coast Clinic staff talked with colleagues currently involved in quality improvement (QI) programs. They reported several shortcomings, including:

- No game plan. Without a way to integrate the quality process with business goals, the quality effort was scattershot and lacked relevance to the organization as a whole. Employees learned QI techniques but had no infrastructure allowing them to use the technique.

- Insufficient physician involvement. Lack of physician participation meant playing with "half a team."

- Train and drain. Employee quality training was wasted when it was not put to immediate and relevant use.

- Lack of accountability. Without clearly assigned responsibilities, employees faltered in their QI efforts. The absence of a quality process leader often meant the collapse of the program.

- Quality "show dogs." Isolated improvements looked good but did not significantly affect quality in ways that mattered to the entire organization. Small successes were common, but significant breakthroughs were rare.

Identifying Key Processes

After investigating some well-known QI consulting firms, the clinic decided to retain a consultant experienced in process management, a systematic approach to QI developed in industry. This approach assumes that processes, not people, are the problem. Process management is an objective methodology that focuses on the actual work that gets done in an organization, breaking down each process into specific activities that can be analyzed and measured. Process management has an impressive track record in manufacturing, but the question in this case was, would it work in a medical clinic?

Using a proprietary methodology called Customer Process Deployment, the consultant helped the clinic develop an organizationwide plan to improve its processes. This approach provided West Coast with a game plan, rather than just a playbook. The "plays" of QI are fairly familiar; statistical process control methods and Pareto diagrams are examples. But actual improvements in quality require a game plan that fits the plays into an overall strategy.

The clinic's strategists, meeting weekly for one-and-a-half hours as the executive quality council, included seven senior administrators, all reporting to the CEO, and five executive physicians. The consultant acted as coach to the council, providing hands-on training in process management techniques.

The council's first task was to determine which processes would help achieve the clinic's overall goal of high quality patient care. Since the patient is the ultimate judge of quality, this task involved viewing the clinic's processes from a patient's point of view. Putting themselves in the patient's shoes, council members mentally toured the clinic, identifying each process a patient encounters. A patient calling to make an appointment, for example, encounters the process "Schedule Patients." The council spent its first two meetings identifying various processes affecting the patient's perception of quality, processes considered central to the clinic's long-term success.

Having identified these key processes, the council created a flowchart of them and their interrelationships. They added support processes as well, those that maintain the processes directly related to patient care. (See Figure 1.) The flowchart represented the entire organization in terms of its processes so people could see how they fit in.

For each box on the chart, a process improvement team was appointed, led by one or more "owners" from the executive quality council. Thus, the chart served as both an organizationwide plan and a management tool for administering that plan.

Selecting a Process to Improve
and Assigning Ownership

The clinic couldn't, of course, improve all of its processes at once; it had to assign priorities to them. The council knew that some processes were working

Figure 1.   Key Processes, West Coast Clinic

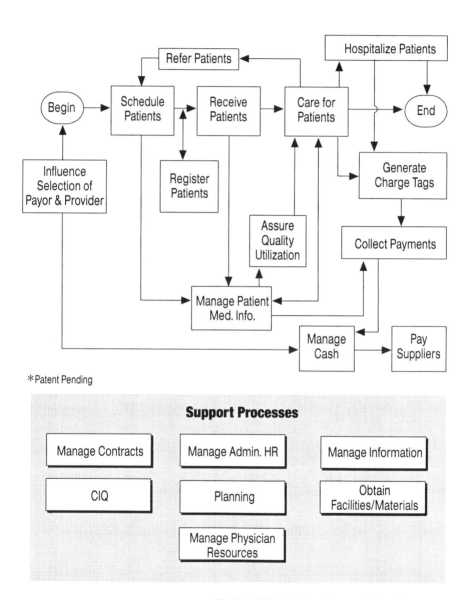

*Patent Pending

well already; others, they knew, had problems, such as the Schedule Patients process. The council chose to focus on this process early on, chiefly because it was an "upstream" process. Errors in an "upstream" process are repeated in subsequent processes, for a costly cascading effect.

The council considered the Schedule Patients process so important that the clinic director and the physician executive director agreed to lead its improvement effort as process co-owners. Assigning ownership to a process builds in accountability and ensures the commitment of top management. Other members of the Schedule Patients process improvement team were the medical director, the clinical area manager, four other physicians, two other administrators, a receptionist, and a facilitator.

The importance of facilitators is worth emphasizing. Facilitators do not need to come from outside the organization, but they should be trained and without a vested interest in the issues under discussion. The clinic's consultant and its director of quality management acted as its first facilitators. They in turn trained other managers to facilitate improvement teams outside their organizational jurisdictions.

Creating the Customer-Supplier Diagram

The first step in improving any process involves identifying the "customers" of the process and the outputs they require from "suppliers." The patient is clearly a customer, but the team spent a considerable amount of time discussing whether or not the physician was a customer of the process, concluding finally that the physician was a supplier of skills and resources to the process, not a customer. An exception was a physician who referred a patient to another physician. In this instance, the referring physician was deemed a customer.

Next, the team identified the measures that process customers use to evaluate quality. Quality measures fell into two categories: cycle time (i.e., the time it takes customers to receive what they request) and adverse indicators (i.e., the customer's negative experiences).

The team agreed that the main cycle time measures were:

- The amount of time spent making the appointment
- Access time, or the time between the making of the appointment and being seen by the physician
- The time between the scheduled appointment hour and when the physician actually sees the patient.
- The adverse indicators for the process included:
- The number of failed attempts to make an appointment
- The number of complaints
- The number of patient "no-shows"

- The number of errors in recording patient information
- The number of patients double-booked at the last minute because the schedule was full

Once the quality measures were identified, the team brainstormed the inputs needed for the Schedule Patients process. The team agreed that the most important input was dependable physician availability to patients. If physicians were seeing too many patients, cycle times were too long. The medical skill mix available had a similar effect. Other factors were available space and equipment, and hours of operation.

At this point, the executive quality council and the process improvement team were ready to create a customer-supplier diagram for the Schedule Patients process. This diagram summarized the customer and supplier inputs, the process outputs, and the quality measures used to evaluate the process, as shown in Figure 2. (A customer-supplier diagram is developed for each key process, as it becomes a candidate for improvement.)

Developing the customer-supplier diagram had several beneficial results. For one thing, staff changed the way they thought about their jobs. They looked at the process objectively, in terms of its activities, and gained an understanding of how their jobs fit into the clinic's overall operations. They also realized that they were working for the patient, not the physician. By taking the patient's viewpoint, the team focused on the appropriate activities to improve. The diagram also clarified responsibility and accountability for the specific activities of the process and established the parameters for analyzing and collecting data.

Identifying What to Improve

To decide what needed improvement, the team created a flowchart of the Schedule Patients process, showing activities and relationships. Examining the process in this new way revealed dozens of opportunities for improvement. Next, the team reviewed the feedback measures — cycle times and adverse indicators — which generated even more ideas for ways to improve. Many improvements involved small changes that the team was able to implement right away, such as using an existing "advice nurse" group in the family practice department to speed the response to patients' messages. It was not always necessary for the entire process team to work on an improvement either; individuals or small subteams could be assigned to various tasks. The more significant projects, however, needed to be explored in more detail.

For example, the team determined that patient no-shows were a significant adverse indicator. The team brainstormed the reasons why a patient might fail to show up for an appointment and charted them on a cause-and-effect diagram. The cause-and-effect diagram then served as a guide in developing a series of open-ended questions for a telephone survey of no-show patients,

Figure 2.   Schedule Patients Process: Customer-Supplier Diagram

Cycle time measure(s):   Access time, time required to schedule an appointment, actual vs. scheduled appointment time

Adverse Indicators: # Patient and referring MD complaints, # no-shows, # incorrect scheduling entries, # access failures, # uninformed patients, # double bookings

Other quality measures: Patient satisfaction level

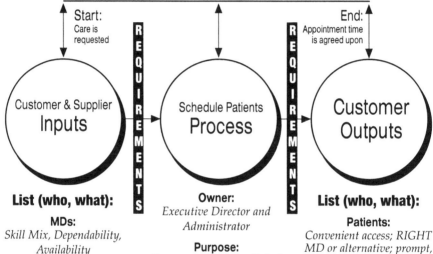

Improvement Team members:

- *medical director*
- *head of nursing*
- *a family practice MD*
- *a department chair*
- *a specialist MD*
- *a receptionist supervisor*
- *a nurse manager*

and the answers to the questions were tallied and graphed on a Pareto diagram.

As Figure 3 shows, the most common reason for no-shows was that the patient forgot about the appointment. To address this problem, the team designed three different reminder systems and is currently measuring test results to determine which works best. Other causes will be addressed as the team's work progresses.

Developing a Review Process

To evaluate improvements and goals, the executive quality council set up a biannual review for each key process. Objective feedback measures include a storyboard display of improvement data (e.g., how much cycle times have been reduced, how many complaints have been received). The quality council also adopted a six-level rating scheme to monitor and evaluate progress. Each rating level has specific requirements that must be met before a process advances to the next highest rating.

In addition to establishing objective measurements of improvement, the review process provides an opportunity to recognize the contributions of team members, boosting morale and team spirit. People feel they have a personal connection to the organization, and that they are helping to make things better. The review process is also a chance to gain executive buy-in for any potentially controversial improvements.

Figure 3.   Pareto Diagram

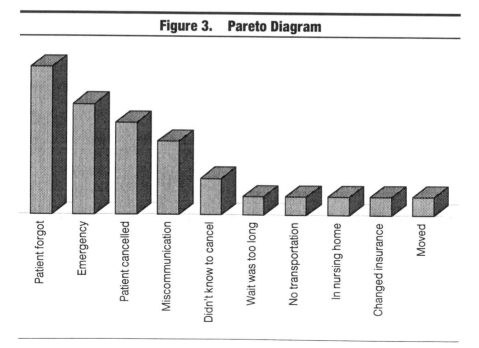

Some Results

In the first year, West Coast Clinic chose four processes to improve: Schedule Patients, Register Patients, Enter Charges, and Manage Patient Medical Information. Results became apparent in only four months. For example, the number of charge sheets turned in by physicians by deadline improved 25 percent, for substantial savings. Claims denials due to registration errors decreased by 50 percent. This gain represented numerous small improvements, but larger gains resulted from single changes, too.

This was the case in pediatrics, which had the longest average waiting room time in the clinic — 30 minutes. The team traced the source of the problem to same-day appointments that were being shoehorned into the schedule. Upon analysis, it turned out that the number of same-day appointments on any given day was predictable. By allowing a certain number of slots for them, the team reduced the 30-minute wait to 19 minutes, a 33 percent improvement.

Results like these have had a favorable effect on the clinic's financial position, but benefits not so easily expressed in percentages have been equally important. One such benefit is the development of in-house management resources. The members of the executive quality council have gained new process management skills that they can use in a variety of situations. And gradually, they are sharing their skills with other managers, as more and more key processes become part of the CQI program and other personnel become involved.

Positive employee relations and an emerging culture of cooperation have been two other results. The objective approach to processes, and not people, minimizes finger pointing, personality conflicts, and attitude problems. People from different departments working as a team get to know one another and form relationships, fostering cooperation. Because everyone on the team has an equal voice, everyone is a stakeholder.

Perhaps the most important benefit of all is that the clinic is seeing improved results all the time. The "continuous" in continuous quality improvement is real.

Lessons Learned

The Customer Process Deployment method the staff used for the West Coast Clinic CQI program avoided the shortcomings colleagues reported at the outset. The clinic learned some important lessons. One was that success depends on understanding the key processes of one's organization. A good rule of thumb is, don't try to improve anything unless you can identify the process to be improved and the specific measure that will signify improvement. A QI strategy based on key processes is a game plan that encompasses the entire organization and ensures significant and relevant results. The structure the clinic chose enabled the clinic to direct the techniques of QI to best advantage.

Linking CQI to the existing management structure also builds in accountability and executive commitment. West Coast Clinic learned that the education of top administrative and physician managers in quality principles and techniques is essential for their participation and follow-through, two critical factors for long-term success.

Coaching proved a very effective way to educate. People learn best by doing. As more and more process improvement teams form, more and more people gain QI skills. And they learn these skills just in-time to put them to use before they are half-forgotten.

Involving the physicians is an ongoing challenge for the clinic. Their attendance at weekly meetings is a significant and essential commitment and the attendance is always better when the issue is one in which they are invested. Here, the key process flowchart itself has proved helpful. When the physicians see how their activities fit into the clinic's game plan, they become more interested in "playing." Sometimes the clinic offers them choices, pointing out the importance of their participation in several processes and asking them to choose the one that appeals to them the most.

Conclusion

In developing a game plan based on key processes, the clinic developed a management system and culture that allow it to improve quality effectively, on a continuous basis. A new rigor of thinking directs the CQI effort, which features objective feedback measures and success indicators that can be compared with benchmarks throughout the industry.

The Customer Process Deployment method worked for West Coast Clinic, and it may work for other medical groups, as well. The industry has a tremendous opportunity to improve processes generic to all clinics — patient registration, scheduling, charts, and many others. For West Coast Clinic, improving key processes has been the most effective way to improve quality, and improving quality is the best way the clinic knows to become a competitive, low-cost provider of first-rate health services.

Questions for Discussion

1. Would these steps work in a smaller group practice? If not, how would you modify the program to provide a better fit?

2. Define continuous quality improvement.

3. What is the role of the facilitator on a CQI team?

4. When implementing a CQI program, why is it so important to define who the customer is?

5. What are the primary reasons that CQI programs fail? That they succeed?

Management of
Human Resources

CASE 11

Conflict in the Anesthesia Associates Group

by Carl Bellas

Anesthesia Associates Group (AAG) is an anesthesia group practice located in a major city. The administrator of the group is Ellen Leslie. After completing her bachelor's degree in nursing, she worked as a critical care nurse in a large hospital and as a nursing administrator. Ms. Leslie then moved to a position as assistant administrator at a large multispecialty clinic and completed her master's degree in health care administration while she continued to work.

Now at AAG, she realizes the extent of the competitiveness of the health care providers market in the city and the effect competition is having and will have on her group's practice. She is concerned that AAG's physicians do not comprehend the serious threats to their futures posed by changes in the national and local health care environments. Ms. Leslie sees very little involvement among the physicians either in the affairs of the group or in the health care system.

The Group

AAG employs 35 anesthesiologists, nine certified registered nurse anesthetists, three clinical support staff, and 12 administrative staff. The group has a contract to provide anesthesia and pain management services to Community Hospitals (CH), a three-hospital system. Approximately one-third of the clinical staff has been with AAG for four years or less, the result of some replacements and some growth. As a hospital-based specialty, the group does not admit patients to the hospital and depends on the surgeon community and Community Hospitals to attract patients for its services.

The group is legally organized as a corporation. Eight of the group's physicians serve as directors, and four of these directors are officers of the corporation and constitute the executive committee.

The Environment

The health care market in the city and adjacent communities is extremely competitive. In addition to CH, there is another three-hospital system, a university teaching hospital, and a large multispecialty group practice. Each of the two private hospital systems is associated with a different managed care program, which results in intense market share competition for the same patient population.

AAG is the only hospital-based anesthesia group in the area providing services as a private practice group. Competition for anesthesia services comes from the physicians employed by the large, multispecialty group practice, the house staff at the university hospital, and a group of individual "partnerships" who share billing services. Three independent anesthesiologists also provide services to Community Hospitals.

A key component of CH's competitive strategy is the organization of the Physician Network, now in its fourth year. The network is designed to increase the hospitals' ability to negotiate arrangements to increase its market share. The network provides a dedicated referral base for the hospitals. CH can contract on behalf of the network physicians through various participation agreements including contracts for services, management agreements, and employment agreements.

The Physician Network was initially formed with primary care physicians. Substantial CH resources were redirected from the enhancement of subspecialties to primary care. Many of the specialty physicians don't understand why CH has changed its historical ways of operating and allocating resources.

The competitive pressures on CH and its responses to them have raised major concerns at AAG. The physicians find themselves facing intense competition from other specialties for hospital resources. They see other group practices being acquired by hospitals and fear becoming hospital employees. They believe that the negotiation of an exclusive contract with CH would be a desirable arrangement for AAG.

Inside the Group

Shortly after assuming her position as administrator, Ms. Leslie met with every member of the group practice. Looking ahead to making recommendations to the officers and the board, she summarized the information she obtained from her meetings.

The physicians' expectations and wishes with respect to workload and income distribution are becoming more diverse. Some of the younger male physicians entered practice with a large student debt and plans to start a family and purchase a home. They want to increase their compensation. The younger female physicians with families want flexible work hours and more time off. In some cases, they have a second income source. Some of the older physicians wish to work more to increase their compensation, while others are willing to reduce their compensation in return for free time and flexibility.

A number of physicians, board members and others, recognize the importance of CH's success to the success of their group. Although AAG is small in numbers, it is a critical part of the hospital system as a whole, and AAG should actively support CH in its efforts.

Almost all of the physicians are dissatisfied with the decision-making process within the organization. The board makes decisions with incomplete information, so that after decisions are made, subsequent information or objections from others in the organization result in the revision or reversal of decisions. This frustrates the board members and causes physicians and staff employees to lose trust in AAG's leadership.

Morale throughout the organization is poor. The issues described above decrease cohesiveness. There is very little interaction among AAG physicians. While most are concerned about the changing nature of health care and their role in it, few are willing to come forward to provide leadership. Beyond the core of active physician participants, the large majority of the physicians either are content to provide anesthesia services or wait to be asked to become involved.

Actions

Ms. Leslie is aware that her personal success and that of AAG depend on increasing the involvement and participation of most of the physicians and the other employees. The traditional dual structure of administrators and physicians is obsolete and not appropriate in the present environment. The inequities in accepting responsibility have to be changed. If AAG is going to accommodate the differing workload and compensation goals of the physicians, then a completely new approach to these issues is needed, and this approach has to be accepted by all. Rather than being merely reactive to competitive pressures in the environment, more of their physicians have to get involved in the discussions that will lead to decisions at CH.

Ms. Leslie presented the board with the summaries of her staff meetings, together with the recommendation that the board work with her to design a strategy to increase physician awareness through education and involvement in the group's planning process. The strategy has to support the participation of the group in the Physician Network and lead to a proactive approach to ensuring AAG's future.

Making participation mandatory is unlikely to be successful, yet the current level of participation is inadequate. The only alternative seems to be to encourage increased participation by improving communication and restructuring the group's decision-making processes.

Ms. Leslie has convinced the board to schedule a retreat with the goal of developing a process that will improve communication and participation. She has arranged for an outside facilitator to lead discussions at the retreat so that she and several other administrators can participate in the discussions.

Questions for Discussion

1. Why are AAG physicians and other physicians hesitant to become involved in decision making and planning in their organizations?

2. Participation may be taking time away from providing income-producing anesthesia services. If a physician serves on boards or committees or in associations that are considered important to AAG, how should his or her compensation reflect the service? What about the potential inequities in workload this might create?

3. Is it possible to offer the physicians a "portfolio" arrangement, whereby individuals make differing contributions to the group?

4. Is the lack of physician involvement serious enough to be considered a competitive weakness?

5. Is Ms. Leslie's focus on changing the manner in which the group plans, makes decisions, and involves its physicians appropriate?

6. What action plans might the board develop at the upcoming retreat?

Practical and Disastrous Applications of Idealism in Human Resources

by Christine Hurley

These are three anecdotes from an experienced executive: my mother taught me that repetition was the key to learning. Throughout my career as a health care administrator, I have found myself rediscovering my basic beliefs and assumptions about the human capacity to make sound decisions about one's own abilities, career, and life. However, there is nothing like a bad burn in the crucible of working with other human beings to make one reexamine one's faith in others. Consider these scenarios:

Scenario 1

Roberta was fresh out of a prestigious Midwest graduate program in public health when she applied for a reception position in a community health clinic. I questioned the match of the position with her interests and abilities, but she was passionate and persuasive in making her case to win the job. She wanted to be part of an organization that really served people in need. With reservations, I hired her. I believed she understood the implications of her choice and could make a better decision for herself than I could.

In the ensuing months, she showed little aptitude for the important interpersonal communications aspects of the job. She also grew restive with the lack of prestige of her job title. She proposed a snappy title change with larger responsibilities. I was increasingly aware that she was unable to perform the core responsibilities of the job. I struggled with the decision to tell her that "this is not working out," while she dreamed of bigger things.

Scenario 2

Oren was a relative star in a field with little competition. As a department manager in a 150-bed hospital within a large staff-model HMO, his reputation was based more on the relative incompetence of his organizational counterparts than on his own real ability and effort. While he was bright, his need for personal recognition usually prevented him from working as an effective member of any team outside of his department.

Despite my poor assessment of his performance, he still carried a positive reputation within the organization and had difficulty accepting my evaluative comments. He believed that he was destined for bigger and better things, yet was unsuccessful in several applications for internal promotions. After several frank, but kind, discussions, we mutually agreed that he would be better off leaving the organization rather than just holding his current place. In an attempt to be supportive of his decision to leave, I negotiated a generous six-month timeline for his departure, including 60 days of special project work. Following his formal announcement to leave, his interest and attention to department management declined radically. He never completed his final project.

Scenario 3

Mark became the program manager in a newly developed hospice facility. In a pressured situation of early organizational startup, I offered the important leadership position to him without an external candidate search. A rapid decision was necessary to maintain momentum after an unexpected separation with the original program manager. Staff were floundering without direction; monumental organizational development lay ahead. Mark's references cautioned me about his shortcomings in the face of conflict, but given his clear strengths in other areas and without a viable alternative, we forged ahead.

In the next months, Mark's strengths as a systematic thinker and teacher were evident, but so were his inadequacies in developing standards of performance, building teams, and confronting the inevitable, unpleasant disciplinary issues. Staff who had come to the new facility with high expectations and idealism became anxious, then angry. They complained they were never invited to be part of decision making as promised, nor were they able to find a means to resolve basic operational questions. Staff registered their problems with the manager, but saw few responses. In the intensity of the operational environment, these shortcomings only added to the grief and emotional exhaustion of the hospice environment.

At first emergence of these problems, I directed staff back to Mark, urging them to try again. They complained that they were not being heard, but dutifully agreed to try. I gave this feedback to Mark at each occurrence, offering advice and support, recognizing all of the work that required his attention, and knowing that everything could not be accomplished at once.

After seven months, and no real improvements, I gave Mark a formal evaluation that credited him with substantial systems progress and also outlined serious concerns about his communications skills and team structure development, and the staff's need for role clarification. Like many employees, he failed to hear the positives and was devastated by the negative feedback in the review. I reiterated my intent to work with him to overcome the issues and to support him in his role. He insisted that he needed my confidence in his abilities. "Was I confident that he could do the job successfully?" I hesitated, feeling caught between the need to be clear that his performance did not meet my expectations and the urge to bolster his resolve and self-confidence. Uneasily, I remarked that I was sure that he could be successful. I wasn't.

The price of "having confidence" in him slowly became obvious. He asked for more time to resolve issues with staff communication. Yet any involvement I had with him on projects was interpreted as a vote of no confidence on my part.

Over the next months, little improvement occurred. In an informal discussion, I asked him if there was anything that I could do to assist him in his work. I reaffirmed my desire that he be successful, and my commitment to support him in his work. He responded by asking why I was unable to say simply that "he was successful," rather than expressing my optimism that he "could be." By external standards, the facility was a success. It had received high praise in an institutional survey process, but the staff concerns were growing. I flinched, feeling boxed-in between the need to be clear and honest about Mark's performance deficits, and the impulse to salvage his self-esteem. Without satisfaction, I told him he was a valuable asset in our success and that we still had many challenges to overcome.

Questions for Discussion

1. How do you balance the need to show respect for the capability and intelligence of people with the occasional need to help them make decisions?

2. What guidelines can be used to determine when you should intervene, and when you should stand back and simply offer support and structured guidance, given an employee who is struggling with significant aspects of performance?

3. What factors should be considered when choosing the specifics of a separation (e.g., severance package, timing)?

4. How would you handle calls from other employers for reference checks on these employees?

PART IV

Practice Management

Group Practice Management and Administration

CASE 13

Restructuring a Joint Venture

by Jerome I. Fink

In 1987, an orthopedic group practice was having difficulty obtaining timely and satisfactory physical therapy treatment for its patients. It was not uncommon for patients to wait two or three weeks for an appointment and then, once the patients were undergoing therapy, communication with their physical therapists was inconsistent. The practice decided to start its own physical therapy clinic, but could not recruit quality therapists because many had what appeared to be an aversion to working for physicians.

One of the practice's physicians had a longstanding friendship with an experienced physical therapist that dated back to their undergraduate days. While this therapist did not want to be an employee of the orthopedic practice, he was comfortable entering into an arrangement with the physicians whereby he could have an ownership interest in the physical therapy clinic. A joint venture arrangement, with the therapist having the minority interest, appeared to be a satisfactory solution for providing the physical therapy required by the practice's patients.

The practice established a new corporation for the sole purpose of operating a physical therapy clinic, and then constructed the clinic. The orthopedic practice physicians, as individuals, owned the majority of the stock in this new corporation and provided all the capital necessary to build and outfit the clinic. Each physician owned an equal share of the majority interest. Although the therapist owned the minority interest, his share was more than twice the size of any one individual physician's share. In addition, the therapist was not required to make a cash contribution, and he did not assume a liability in connection with the clinic. Cash distributions were made on a regular basis to the physicians and the therapist in proportion to their stock ownership.

At the same time, the therapist formed his own independent management company, which provided the physical therapists, assistants, and administrative personnel necessary to operate the clinic. The management company, wholly owned by the therapist, was responsible for hiring, training, and paying all clinic personnel. For its efforts, the management company was paid, by the clinic, a percentage of the clinic's net billings. Further, the contract between the management company and the clinic provided a very generous severance payment to the therapist should the clinic terminate the management company without cause.

The orthopedic practice provided management for all nonphysical therapy activities, and all billing, collections, record-keeping, and bookkeeping functions. For these services, the clinic paid the orthopedic practice a percentage of net billings (less cash collected at the clinic).

Upon advice of legal counsel, the physicians and the physical therapist decided not to refer Medicare patients to the clinic, in order to preclude any possible conflict with the then existing federal rules and regulations. In addition, anticipating governmental changes in the future, the joint venture agreement included the following provision:

> If the basic structure, format, or method of organization of the Corporation or the services supplied by the different parties to the Agreement is found to be in violation of any law or governmental or ethical rule or regulation, the parties will make every reasonable effort to amend this Agreement in a mutually acceptable manner or otherwise restructure the business venture contemplated hereunder so as to preserve the rights, duties, and economic benefits contemplated herein.

For five years, this arrangement was of great benefit to the patients, therapists, and physicians. However, in 1992, introduction of legislation at both state and federal levels threatened the arrangement and caused the practice to begin a comprehensive review of the viability of the joint venture agreement. The following statement, from a piece of legislation introduced by the state's legislative bodies, illustrated the cause for concerns: "physicians should not refer patients to a health care facility outside their office practice at which they do not directly provide care or services when they have an investment interest in the facility." Although this legislation was put aside for the session, there was a promise to reconsider similar legislation in 1993.

And further, as reported in the April 1992 MGMA Update, in an article entitled "Stark Rules on Self-Referrals Issued," the U.S. Congress appears likely to expand the applicability of the self-referral rules beyond laboratory services to imaging, physical therapy, and other services at some point in the future; and states are considering laws similar to the Stark bill with applicability, in some cases, to all payers. State legislatures are likely to borrow detailed definitions and other provisions directly from the federal regulations. The article continued, "Perhaps of biggest concern, the proposal provides no grace period for those who may need to restructure existing arrangements based on regulatory provisions that should have been disseminated before rather than after the January 1 effective date" (Saner 1992).

Upon completion of the review of the joint venture agreement, and after obtaining legal advice, the practice came to the conclusion that the joint venture should be terminated before legislation was enacted that would severely limit or prohibit referrals and thereby diminish the value of the physicians' investment. The date for termination was set at, on, or before December 31, 1992. This date was considered significant because of the possibility that the above-reported state legislation would be passed in the spring of 1993 and made retroactive to January 1, 1993. Four alternative actions were considered.

1. Sell the physical therapy clinic to the minority-interest therapist.
2. Sell the physical therapy clinic to some outside source.
3. Purchase the minority interest therapist's share of the clinic, merge the clinic into the orthopedic practice, and hire the therapist to manage the clinic.
4. Purchase the minority interest therapist's share of the clinic, merge the clinic into the orthopedic practice, and hire some other physical therapist to manage the clinic.

Three of the practice's physicians were assigned to function as a negotiations committee and directed to meet with the therapist to determine his views and then to make recommendations to the group. The therapist's physician friend, who at this time was the incumbent practice president, excluded himself from the committee because he believed he could not be objective. The practice administrator did not participate in the discussions because the physical therapist wanted the discussions to be limited to health care professionals.

Discussions between the negotiations committee and the therapist began in February, and it was evident from the beginning that the therapist did not share the physicians' view that action had to be taken to terminate the joint venture prior to the end of 1992. The therapist assured the negotiations committee that, if legislation should ever be enacted that would prohibit or severely handicap the existing agreement, he would, at that time, purchase the physical therapy clinic for a fair price.

Since selling the clinic to the therapist was already the first choice of the physicians, the discussions were then focused on convincing the therapist that sale of the clinic had to be accomplished in 1992 and on determining the selling price.

However, during the meetings that took place in the months of March and April, the therapist continued to insist that there was no need for him to purchase the clinic in 1992. Rather than discuss the timing of the sale, the therapist introduced information he had gathered that showed that he was responsible for generating a larger part of the clinic's business than that for which he was given credit and that his affiliation with the orthopedic practice was actually costing him revenue. The therapist's conclusions were not supported by the objective information that the practice administrator made available to the physicians.

By May, the negotiations committee finally succeeded in convincing the therapist that he had to decide whether or not he would buy the physical therapy clinic. With the purchase price yet to be decided, the therapist then informed the committee that he could not purchase the clinic in one lump sum, but would have to buy it in installments. The negotiations committee sought legal advice and was told that, in the opinion of the corporate attorney, an installment sale could be considered a violation of the self-referral statutes inasmuch as it could be seen that the physicians were referring patients to the clinic so that the therapist would be able to make the installment payments. Thus, after three months of discussions, the option of selling the clinic to the therapist had to be discarded.

The negotiations committee and the therapist then began discussions on the physicians' second choice, that is, purchasing the therapist's interest in the clinic, merging the clinic into the orthopedic practice, and hiring the therapist to manage the physical therapy portion of the orthopedic practice.

In June, the therapist was offered an employment agreement that guaranteed him the same compensation he enjoyed with the management company; a lump-sum purchase of his stock in the clinic; a bonus designed to pay him the same amount of money he would have received if he had been able to maintain his minority interest; and a severance payment (if terminated without cause) identical to the one that had been in his management company agreement.

In all respects, this financial offer was as good as, or better than, the arrangement that was then in effect. The only drawback was that the therapist would no longer be an owner. The therapist said that he thought the offer was fair.

Two weeks later, without commenting on the new employment offer, the therapist sent a letter to the negotiations committee stating that he had been underpaid for the last five years because the formula used to compute payments to the management company was at variance with the 1987 contract. In fact, the contract had erroneously used the term "net billings" in place of the term "net charges." Once again the practice consulted legal counsel. Subsequently, all of the practice physicians, the therapist, and the practice administrator met. It was pointed out to the therapist that the corporate attorney had included in his 1987 notes that the computation formula was explained in detail to the therapist and that "net billings" referred to "net." The practice administrator reminded the therapist that, from the very beginning of clinic operations, he and the therapist had jointly reviewed the monthly payment calculations and had never found a discrepancy. The therapist withdrew his complaint.

In July, the negotiations committee again met with the therapist to discuss the employment agreement. The therapist stated that the agreement was all right; however, he now questioned the charges attributed to billing and administration. He wanted to reduce the payments made to the orthopedic practice for billings, which would have the effect of increasing his bonus. Furthermore, he decided that he should receive a higher percentage of the physical therapy net charges.

All of the practice physicians met to discuss the negotiations and concluded that the therapist was not negotiating in good faith. The majority of the physicians now believed that the therapist would do whatever was necessary to prolong the negotiations process. His goal appeared to be to delay merging the clinic into the orthopedic practice until 1993 when he would have a chance, if passage of state law made it illegal for the physicians to continue their ownership interest, to purchase the physical therapy clinic at a bargain price. Accordingly, the negotiations chairman was to move ahead cordially, but firmly, and get the employment contract signed and the management contract terminated.

The negotiations committee chairman notified the therapist that the proposed employment offer would not be altered. The therapist, stating that he still had some questions, requested that his lawyer be present at the next meeting. The chairman agreed, with the understanding that the practice administrator would also attend.

The next meeting was held in September, and the negotiations committee, practice administrator, therapist, and therapist's attorney were present. The attorney had prepared a long list of questions relating to the proposed employment agreement for the therapist. One by one, the physicians and practice administrator responded to the queries. After about 90 minutes, the attorney turned to the therapist and said, "You've got a good deal here. I recommend that you sign this agreement." The impasse appeared to be over.

The negotiations committee chairman then carefully explained that the current management contract with the therapist required a 90-day termination notice and, accordingly, written notice would be sent to the therapist prior to October 1. The therapist and his attorney said that this was not a problem, for the employment agreement was going to be signed. Written termination of the management contract was hand delivered to the therapist on September 24.

In the first week of October, the negotiations committee chairman, practice administrator, and therapist met for what was understood to be the signing of the employment agreement. The therapist, saying that he had changed his mind, would not sign the agreement. The negotiations committee chairman asked the therapist if he knew when he had decided not to sign the agreement? The therapist replied that he had never intended to sign an employment agreement, for he did not wish to be an employee of physicians. Thus, negotiations with the therapist were ended.

The physicians' third-choice alternative was to sell the physical therapy clinic to some outside source. After considering the number of days available to consummate a sale, (fewer than 90), and the reality of contending with a lame-duck clinic manager, the physicians decided to pursue the fourth-choice alternative, that is, to purchase the minority interest therapist's share of the clinic, merge the clinic with the orthopedic practice, and hire some other physical therapist to manage the clinic. Accordingly, the physicians bought the minority interest therapist's share of the clinic on December 1, and on December 31 the clinic was merged into the orthopedic practice.

Also, on December 1, the minority interest therapist told his employees that he was going to terminate them in 30 days. A meeting was arranged with the physical therapy clinic employees and the orthopedic practice administrator, at which a very candid conversation was held. The physical therapy clinic personnel were advised of many of the details of the failed negotiations with the clinic manager and told that it was the clinic manager's decision not to be an employee of the physicians. They were also told that the physicians desired to continue clinic operations with no change in the manner that patients were being treated. The end result was that all clinic personnel opted to remain as employees of the orthopedic practice, and the assistant clinic manager was promoted to clinic manager.

It has been two years since the former clinic manager, and minority interest owner, has departed, and the physical therapy clinic continues to be of great benefit to the practice's patients, therapists, and physicians.

This whole experience has taught the practice a number of lessons which include:

- Legal contracts should be complete and all provisions and projections fully and carefully analyzed. The therapist's management contract provided for a severance payment in the event the therapist was terminated without cause. This payment clause was for the therapist's protection, and all that was considered was the minimum sum the therapist would receive if terminated without cause. However, the clinic's financial success was much greater than originally anticipated, and this gave rise to a very large severance payment for without-cause termination, which may have materially influenced the therapist's decisions.

- Legal contracts should contain the final agreed-upon language. Using the term "net billings" instead of what was really meant, "net charges" caused unnecessary meetings and increased legal fees. The assumption that what is in the contract does not matter, since all parties to the contract are friends anyway, may not hold.

- The most qualified individuals should be assigned to the negotiations committee.

- The practice attorney should be included in the negotiations process from the very beginning.

- A realistic timetable should be set for actions to be taken and, if possible, all the negotiating participants should concur with it.

- Each negotiations meeting needs a prepared agenda, and each item on the list should be reviewed prior to the introduction of new issues.

Questions for Discussion

1. What are the major steps in preparing for the negotiations process?
2. What could the administrator have done to conclude negotiations in a more timely fashion?
3. Discuss the implications of the Stark legislation on other relationships in the group practice setting.
4. What outside resources could the clinic administrator have used to help resolve the problem?
5. Identify the key issues associated with absorbing the employees of the physical therapy clinic into the orthopedic group practice setting?

Reference

Saner, R. J. 1992. "Stark Rules on Self-Referrals Issued." *MGMA Update* 31(4): 125.

CASE 14

The Dark Side of Physician Compensation

by Steven Paul Fiore

The physicians and management of Orthopedic Group, Inc. (OGI) have expended more time and energy on physician compensation systems than on any other single management problem. No matter what the operational issue or the product development strategy being considered, the ultimate determining factor is always, how will the cash be distributed?

Since the establishment of this single-specialty medical practice in the early 1970s, the compensation system has been based on "equal distribution." Regardless of the distribution of workload, all physicians have shared equally in the economic rewards of the practice.

However, as original members aged and younger, more specialty-trained physicians joined the group, workloads became significantly unbalanced. In addition, shareholder physicians started to drift away from full-time, practice-oriented activities. Some of their endeavors were in associated businesses that did not contribute any income to the practice or offset any physician-related expenses.

The younger and more productive physicians became increasingly disenchanted with "carrying" the physicians who chose to slow down or alter their practice activities. As the group size increased, the amount of cash available for distribution grew as well. The equal-share formula was no longer acceptable and resulted in a management controversy over the merits of the practice's compensation system.

Background and Scope

Practice Configuration

OGI is structured as a professional service corporation directed by a four-member board of directors. Each board member is an equal shareholder in the corporation.

The group has expanded from four to seven physicians, and the current physician mix includes fellowship-trained spine surgery and sports medicine specialists along with general orthopedists. The board has always recognized and accepted the fact that revenue production is influenced by a physician's specific subspecialty, but has also maintained the premise that equal-share income distribution is best for the practice.

Prior to 1988, the group experienced little physician expansion. Two of the original shareholders were approaching their middle sixties, and a third was in his late fifties. Associate physicians joined the practice slowly, under extremely controlled arrangements, usually as older physicians were preparing to retire.

The definition of retirement was also a problem. The original shareholders' agreements contained provisions that, after a certain age, physicians could elect to stop taking night call and reduce their work hours, yet retain their equal share of the corporation. Unfortunately, all of the original shareholders aged together, which meant that recruitment became critical to perpetuating the group.

The odds of successful recruitment were enhanced by OGI's reputation and command of the marketplace. As a result, the practice was able to add four new physicians in six years, but this resulted in a disproportionate mix of physicians by age. This, combined with the subspecialty interests and fellowship training, set the stage for dissatisfaction with the income-distribution arrangement.

The group has a 50 percent overhead factor and continues to base all compensation on this value. Practice values for buy-in and buy-out are determined annually by the practice's independent, certified public accounting firm. In addition to the book value of the corporation, the buy-out includes a predetermined amount of the specific physician's accounts receivable, but the buy-in does not include accounts receivable or goodwill. During new group members' two-year period as associate physicians, their salary is fixed and guaranteed. The two-year employment period in essence funds the buy-in via production surplus going to the shareholders. This method has kept the buy-in relatively low, and reasonably affordable for young physicians.

The accounts payable system absorbs and pays operating expenses and other overhead-related expenditures. Bonus dollars are subject to overhead modifications in order to account for both work and expense variations that occur throughout the fiscal year.

The financial health of the group had reached an awkward stage. Managed care had made a solid penetration in OGI's marketplace, which resulted in numerous reductions in reimbursements. As with any business, once rev-enue becomes restricted, other associated problems occur. The practice was able to maintain salaries and meet its expense liabilities; however, a smaller pool of bonus dollars remained.

Expenses did not rise, but the overhead percentage did increase due to the reduction in revenues. The medical staff were made aware that this percentage was a mathematical relationship of revenue to expenses. Nevertheless, the younger physicians felt that the equal-distribution system made unfair demands on them.

As the dynamics of OGI changed and the effects of managed care and gen-eral changes to the economy permeated the practice, income became less predictable. For years, the physicians had reviewed the daily charges and drawn conclusions about their income levels. Expenses and overhead were addressed through accounting reports, and no one paid much attention to them. There seemed to be a never-ending supply of patients and revenue.

Now, however, the group's viability was at stake. Maintaining order and group integrity would require innovative strategic solutions. OGI needed to explore contractual relationships with third-party carriers, do a better job of forecasting patient volume, review expense categories, and generally operate more efficiently. The most difficult task, though, would be to redesign physi-cian compensation. This being the most sensitive issue, required participation by the physicians and a fair amount of finesse. Physician paranoia would surely scuttle this process.

Compensation Structure

OGI is a Subchapter S professional service corporation It uses a cash-method accounting system with biweekly payroll. The shareholders receive a regular, predetermined salary. Bonuses, if any, are distributed annually. The associate physicians have a salary schedule governed by contract.

The practice tinkered with compensation mechanisms for several years, but it stopped short of developing a thorough, well-thought-out process to maximize personal physician income. Generally, nothing changed except the amount of salary paid for a particular fiscal year.

This method worked fine until 1987, when the practice expanded to a new physical plant. The physicians planned and executed this expansion without the assistance of a practice administrator. They underestimated the cost of the project, and the resulting debt service was substantial. At the same time, one of the older shareholders announced his retirement, which placed further bur-dens on the younger physicians.

Given the state of OGI's financial affairs, several of the younger sharehold-ers believed that the group needed a professional administrator to manage the practice and lead the corporation into the future. They advocated for this posi-tion successfully, and by the end of the administrator's first fiscal year, the board of directors finally had good financial information available to use in setting salary levels and evaluating compensation systems.

In each of the fiscal years 1989, 1990, 1991, and 1992, the board of directors elected to raise salary levels. Operations from those fiscal years resulted in substantial bonuses. However, this disbursement was still based on an equal compensation system.

The associate physicians contributed to the revenue pool, but played little role in determining compensation structure. They did, however, make their personal feelings about it known.

Defining what constituted compensation was a difficult undertaking. Referring to the physicians' W2 statements was misleading and not conclusive. The shareholders had strange habits of buying items and billing these purchases to the office. The company became responsible for these acquisitions, and treated them as a pretax benefit. OGI could never reach an understanding as to how this mechanism was supposed to work or be monitored. At best, the group attempted to "balance" the value of this benefit at the end of each fiscal year.

In addition to being inequitable, this system was unmanageable; it did not allow the practice to plan for these expenditures. OGI needed an approach that still reimbursed shareholders for their business expenses but allowed the group to budget and plan for these expenses.

For years, the corporation's shareholders met at the end of each fiscal year and decided the amount of funds to be distributed as bonuses. Unfortunately, short-term needs exerted undue influence in this method. The retirement of a shareholder, short-term debt service, pension requirements, or some other expenditure altered the amount of funds available. Although these needs were important, they often developed at the hand of one shareholder and did not have equal importance to all shareholders in the practice. A bonus program needed to be developed that would provide for an attainable reward system at the conclusion of each fiscal year. The plan could not be influenced by short-term needs or personal objectives, or at the overall expense of the corporation.

One last, complicating factor had to do with compensation earned outside the practice. The employment contracts for each physician in the practice prohibited outside employment of any type. Any compensation a physician received from an outside activity was to become the property of the corporation. The practice had developed two subsidiary companies, providing occupational medicine and rehabilitation, and the franchising management systems. Each of these two subsidiary organizations required a commitment of time from an OGI shareholder to assist in its clinical management, and the time these physicians spent on these organizations seriously affected their financial contribution to the corporation.

Scope of the Problem

The older physicians' priorities were changing from work to family. Overall quality of life seemed to be the major goal for these physicians. The younger physicians could not justify the cost placed on them to support this philosophy. The priorities of the younger physicians were to secure their financial future, fund their pensions, and retire their personal medical education debts. For the younger physicians to attain the same financial status as the older physicians would be difficult and would require dramatic changes in the way economic rewards were attained.

Decision and Implementation

Evaluated Financial Goals of the Board of Directors

The board of directors faced the difficult task of assessing the corporation's financial goals while at the same time deciding the financial future of the shareholders. They believed a new risk-based compensation system was the best strategy for the shareholders. This strategy would shift more of the burden for the physician's compensation directly to the physician and away from the corporation. The compensation system for associate physicians would remain unchanged, with one exception. In addition to the fixed salary, a discretionary bonus was introduced, to be based on the shareholders' bonus pool. This would maintain full participation by the associates and remove any risk of poor behavior.

A Set of Criteria to Meet Financial Goals

Criteria were needed to assess this risk-based strategy and determine the amount of compensation the practice could comfortably afford. In addition, an expense program would be considered part of the total compensation package rather than a fiscal year-end exercise.

Minimum patient loads and surgical time access were established. This created production goals for all the physicians. These goals took into consideration vacation allocation and continuing medical education (CME) time. The corporation would not buy back any unused vacation or CME time. OGI felt it was extremely important that all physicians take their vacations in order to separate themselves from the practice and continue their education.

Determining an accurate overhead factor would be critical in this process. Regardless of the final compensation formula, overhead expenses needed to be satisfied before any compensation was paid. The one point of consensus among the board of directors was that overhead would be included in every aspect of the compensation system. OGI's certified public accounting firm recalculated the overhead, and it remained at 50 percent.

Work schedules and operational parameters had to be reestablished for each physician. These new parameters were set by the automated scheduling system, based on the physicians' historical work patterns. Physicians were permitted to customize their schedules to a certain degree. Minimums were established, but individual physicians could expand their patient load or rearrange the timing of the schedule to meet their specific practice needs.

Operating room schedules underwent the most significant changes. Surgeons were no longer allowed to operate in the morning and see office patients in the afternoon. They were given whole days in the operating room rather than half-days. Physician extenders were used to assist in the operating room, rather than tying up a second surgeon.

Night call, vacation time, and CME time were scheduled four months in advance, rather than month-to-month. This allowed the physicians to plan their time better and achieve a more constant flow of patients.

Several modifications were made to the shareholders' employment agreements. The most significant changes related to compensation derived from disability and outside remuneration. The board of directors modified the salary continuation plan by not permitting a disabled physician to be paid a salary while receiving disability payments.

Working for either of the practice's subsidiary organizations would still be considered outside employment. However, before a physician could accept any form of compensation from a subsidiary, the subsidiary would need to pay to the practice the portion of practice overhead attributed to that physician.

The board of directors developed specific guidelines for measuring work and output for each physician. The board became extremely sensitive to any one physician trying to manipulate the system to improve his or her own overall contribution.

Alternative Compensation Plans Considered

A new compensation system had to be developed to resolve the problem of unbalanced compensation. The aging of the shareholders, outside interests, and the unbalanced work production were good indications that the logical solution would be to convert to a straight productivity formula. The biggest problem of shifting to a productivity-based compensation system was that none of the physicians had any experience with the intricacies of this type of system. Developing a formula that properly accounted for overhead, patient mix, payer mix, and cooperation was complicated, if not frightening, to the younger shareholders.

A plan using an equal salary as a base and a bonus system derived from production was considered. This would protect the base salary of the less active shareholder physicians and provide an added income opportunity for higher producers. The mechanism would allow older shareholders to work at a comfortable pace and continue their participation in the related subsidiary organizations.

Rules of operation were needed to ensure that the practice was able to function properly. A minimum number of patient sessions and operative time for each physician was established. These new parameters were created to guarantee the practice the level of patient activity it needed to meet its financial obligations. As part of the rules of operation, the staff had to monitor changes to the schedule to ensure that the minimum requirements were achieved. Any physician reducing or canceling patient sessions had to make them up. Increases to the schedules were permitted, however, not if they imposed on another physician's time or caused the corporation to incur overtime.

Practice dynamics were in a delicate state. With new rules of operation, everyone in the practice had the responsibility to ensure that OGI achieved its goals without sacrificing patient services. The group realized that surgeons feel more productive in the operating room, but the office volume was more valuable in the long term. OGI's ability to make patients happy would be the long-term goal of the practice.

Patient satisfaction was the practice's ultimate goal regardless of the compensation system. Monitoring patient concerns would be as important as resolving patients' medical problems. It was recognized that allowing a physician to shortchange one patient's follow-up visit in order to add a new patient in the schedule, or to keep patients waiting longer because of an extra patient forced into the schedule, would reflect negatively on the whole practice.

Another factor of concern was how the relationship between the shareholder physicians and associate physicians would evolve. As in most practices, OGI's older physicians provide its younger physicians with patients. Each time an associate physician is added to the practice, the shareholders direct a certain number of patients to that associate to help build his or her practice. The total number of patients treated remains the same, but a distinct decline in the shareholder productivity is usually experienced.

Constructing a compensation plan that included characteristics each physician wanted was a formidable task. The established criteria limited options and creativity. The basic components were evident in each version considered; assembling the plan was the real challenge.

The first plan the practice evaluated was a straight salary system. The board of directors proposed to raise the base salary of each shareholder to a level consistent with the AAOS and MGMA tables contained in the 1991 Physician Compensation and Production Survey (Cekja et al. 1991). This would offer the advantage of maintaining the one-for-all philosophy and a simple budget. The distribution system would, however, remain inequitable. The plan would also require OGI to shift certain company-paid pretax benefits back to the individual physicians.

The second plan considered was an equal-salary, equal-bonus, and equal-expense program. It would allocate a fixed amount of money to each shareholder to cover automobile, business, and CME expenses, and dues and subscriptions. Each shareholder would submit a detailed monthly expense report, and receive reimbursement through the normal accounts payable system. The plan would keep salaries lower and manageable from a budget and funding perspective. It did not resolve the problem of the unbalanced workload. However, it would shift more of the economic reward to the fiscal year end, and distribute the cash in the truest sense of a bonus. The other advantage of this plan was the pretax benefit of the expense program. Not only would each physician be able to receive the pretax value of his or her automobile and business expense reimbursement, but the company would be able to budget for these expenses and spread the liability across the entire fiscal year.

The third plan was a production-based system that shifted all of the economic rewards directly to the physicians. This plan was at the opposite end of the spectrum from the first option. The physicians would be paid monthly based on a 50 percent overhead factor. In addition, personal and business expenses would become the physician's own responsibility. The advantage of this plan was that it recognized differences in workload and rewarded the more active physicians. The disadvantage was that the senior members of the group would be severely penalized, possibly giving rise to disruptive behavior. In addition, controversial debates regarding overhead and goodwill were likely to emerge. This certainly would have defeated the fundamental premise of a group practice.

The last option considered was a blend of the other three plans. The plan consisted of a base salary, determined by calculating the average shareholder's production. The salary level would ensure that each physician was reasonably paid for the normal work expectation. The expense program was included, which would give an equal benefit to each shareholder and which was, in essence, funded by a shift in salary dollars. The third component was a bonus, based on a production formula.

This integrated plan protected the senior members and allowed them to maintain a certain quality of life. It addressed workload by putting a portion of income at risk. It allowed the company to maintain the benefit plan and spread the liability across the entire fiscal year. The disadvantage of this system was its direct dependence on company operations. If the company performed poorly, available bonus dollars would not exist, resulting in the potential for a net decrease in compensation. Obviously, this could be expected in any system adopted. With more income at risk, however, the effect could be more severe.

Possible Solutions

The board of directors decided that the inequitable compensation problem was real enough, and that the environment in which the group practiced medicine was only going to become more difficult. To retain a system that was no longer fair or equally beneficial was disruptive and not worth the conflict being generated.

A new compensation system designed on the blended method was introduced for fiscal year 1992. As part of this new plan, it was necessary to revise practice expectations. The physicians had to maintain minimum production targets. In essence, each physician needed to generate two times the value of his or her salary, benefits, and expense program before he or she could participate in any bonus. This ensured that all physicians met their obligations and that the additional economic rewards could only be attained through additional work.

This methodology instilled an entrepreneurial spirit in all of the physicians. They began seeking extra work and completing forms and other related tasks whose failure to be completed had once impeded reimbursement. Each physician identified new priorities and focused more time on the practice and less on outside, non-revenue-producing endeavors. The practice became more aggressive at attracting patients and in managed care arrangements. This paradigm shift in the physician culture fostered more successful long-range planning. The opportunity for non-patient-related income from lectures, publishing, and work with the subsidiary organizations became easier to achieve and less confrontational.

Results and Conclusions

Once the physicians accepted the new business guidelines and were comfortable with how the system functioned, it was easier to schedule patients. As a result, gross revenues for the practice reached an all-time high. Revenues for fiscal year 1992 were $600,000, or 15 percent greater than the previous fiscal year. The shareholders participated in the bonus pool and provided a bonus to the associate physicians. Personal income reached the highest level that any physician had previously experienced.

When this plan was designed, a strategy was established with guidelines that set out group-oriented priorities. These priorities consisted of minimal office disruptions, patient satisfaction, participation in programs that benefited the group, and the flexibility to respond to change. However, as the fiscal year progressed, the physicians increasingly ignored or dismissed the group-oriented priorities in order to pursue personal revenue-generating tasks. Individual goals took priority over the group's objectives. Two of the physicians constantly changed schedules and disrupted the office, canceled meetings, overbooked schedules (causing patient dissatisfaction), and performed procedures they were not accustomed to performing.

Disruptive behavior was not universal among the shareholder physicians. Most of the other shareholder physicians followed the guidelines and complied with the group objectives. One specific physician, however, the one who spent the most time with the subsidiary organizations, became tenacious in his disregard for the productivity system. His flouting of the rules of operation and his self-serving attitude created considerable conflict with his partners and contributed to a general state of tension and disharmony.

This conflict took its toll on OGI employees. They were constantly caught in the middle of trying to cooperate with the instructions of the physicians and, at the same time, trying to adhere to company policy. One physician often humiliated individual secretaries for following the instructions of another physician. Patient complaints increased, and administration could not always resolve them. Staff morale became a serious problem because physician leadership allowed the behavior to persist.

The net result of the system was twofold. First, a point was proved that more work could be accomplished given a direct financial incentive. Second, the physicians of this group were not capable of maintaining the long-standing all-for-one-and-one-for-all relationship that had been the foundation of this organization.

The board of directors determined that the cost of this system was not worth the economic reward it generated. The system was discontinued at the completion of fiscal year 1992. The board reverted back to a compensation plan of equal salary set at a higher level and equal bonus. The expense program was retained and included in the compensation package.

Recommendations

Several mistakes caused the system to fail. First, the board of directors decided to make a wholesale conversion of a very sensitive, complicated system in a relatively short period of time. They should have developed a phase-in methodology or, at least, not had as large a portion of compensation influenced by productivity.

The second mistake was relying on a compensation system to modify physician behavior. Becoming creative is healthy. Making changes that move too far away from traditional expectations, however, can make success very difficult to attain.

The third mistake was not doing an accurate job at forecasting revenue. The year before the system was implemented had a relatively small bonus pool available. The effect of applying the bonus formula to that pool of funds was therefore not significant in relation to total income. However, the change in physician behavior during the first year of implementation of the new plan resulted in such a significant surplus that the available pool of bonus funds nearly matched the base salary for some of the physicians. The board of directors neither anticipated this result nor handled it well.

Finally, OGI failed to protect its staff. The staff were subjected to unacceptable working conditions, and the board of directors provided them with only minimal support or corrective action. The physicians often engaged in their own conflicts in the presence of the staff, which reduced staff effectiveness and weakened morale. The organization lost sight of the fact that the staff were its most valuable resource and failed to respect their feelings and maintain a proper work environment. To compound this problem, the shareholder physicians were setting the tone for the associate physicians, who were developing similar habits. This led to problems as the associates matured through their contract periods to shareholder status.

The board of directors recognized that, even though personal income rose, quality of life and harmony took a precipitous decline, and they were critical to the practice's long-run ability to survive. Although the blended compensation system failed, the practice benefited from updated operating procedures, cost reductions, and exposure to the importance of patient satisfaction. Because practice revenue increased, the board had the luxury of adjusting salaries to maintain physician motivation and ensure participation in corporate goals. The following fiscal year was far less stressful with respect to compensation. The board of directors modified the night call and caseload aspects of shareholder agreements to account for changes in activity. However, the board still will not consider a change from the equal-distribution compensation system.

Questions for Discussion

1. Summarize the reasons why the recommended compensation plan failed.

2. What could the administrator have done differently to reduce the turmoil associated with the change in the compensation system?

3. Would tensions be the same in a nonsurgical group practice?

4. Where would an administrator go to research the question of compensation alternatives?

5. Why were the associates (new physicians in their first two years with the group) unhappy with their compensation system?

6. What are the hazards to the group of placing too much emphasis on pure productivity?

Reference

Center for Research in Ambulatory Health Care Administration, MGMA, in *Physician Compensation Survey*: 1991 Report Based on 1990 Data, p. 24. Cekja & Co., St. Louis, Missouri, provided funding and support for this survey.

CASE 15

Reorganization of a Buy-Sell Agreement

by Chad L. Peter

The group practice was organized as a professional service corporation whose stockholders consisted of the medical physicians. These physicians were also stockholders of an affiliated real estate corporation in which they held majority interest along with a group of dentists and the administrator. When the organization was set up in 1962, it was under the premise that the capital invested in the real estate corporation by each stockholder would appreciate at a rate of 6 to 7 percent a year and would be a form of retirement benefit for each stockholder. This appreciation would be deferred until the stockholder retired or left the group practice.

To support the projected buyouts, the real estate corporation had to show a net profit of approximately $50,000 annually. For the real estate corporation to generate this profit, additional rents and utility payments had to be made by the professional service corporation consisting of the group physicians. At this time, the group was in a growth phase and needed all of the capital to support its cash flow. The professional service corporation had been running in a deficit operating position and had tax credits to use, whereas the real estate corporation was operating at a profit level and was paying taxes. This caused a conflicting problem in that the professional service corporation was depleting its net profits to support the growth of the real estate corporation for the future buy-outs.

The physicians felt they were also facing three other large problems with this organizational structure. First, the real estate buy-sell agreement called for a $40,000 buy-in to become a partner in this group. This was becoming a detriment to recruiting new physicians. Because many other group practices were not requiring ownership, the additional debt was scaring away recruits. Changes in the tax law in 1986 affected the interest deductions on investment incomes such as this and made the situation worse for physicians who had to leverage the entire amount. The group felt it needed to lower the buy-in to new physicians, but it placed priority also on maintaining equality among the existing physicians who had invested heavily in the corporation.

The second problem was the unfunded equity in the real estate corporation. The group's organized buy-sell agreement was based on an annual increase in the share value, to be set by the board of directors. The historical increase had been 6 percent per year, tied to the fair market value of the real estate. Based on periodic appraisals by the Member Appraisal Institute (MAI), the plan called for the group to maintain at least a 20 percent equity position in the real estate corporation so that the real estate corporation would never be more than 80 percent leveraged as retirements and buy-outs began to happen. The problem existed in that the plan was not funded. New physicians were being saddled with large retirement debt in order to satisfy the buy-sell agreement.

Third, the banks were evaluating properties such as this one differently. Instead of looking only at the book value of a property, they were also considering the real market value.

Administrative Goals

To get a handle on these problems, the group employed a consultant to evaluate the group's position and, more important, to find out what other group practices were doing. After meeting with the consultant and Wellness Partners' accountant and attorneys, the practice set these goals:

1. Freeze the current equity growth in the real estate corporation.
2. Remove the disincentive to new physicians of a high buy-in.
3. Guarantee fair treatment by recognizing the equity interest of existing shareholders.
4. Avoid significant adverse tax consequences.

After much discussion, the group focused on four alternatives.

Alternative 1. Recapitalization through Stock Exchange

Under Alternative 1, the group practice would issue a new class of preferred stock in exchange for the real estate corporation stock. A dividend would be paid each year on the preferred stock. Each existing physician would maintain $5,000 in voting common stock, and new physicians would buy in at the $5,000 limit. By issuing and transferring the stock, the real estate corporation would be merged into the group practice corporation. This would lower the buy-in amount and freeze the unfunded growth in real estate appreciation. The preferred class of stock would eventually be eliminated through attrition as physicians retired.

Advantages

1. The unfunded growth in the real estate corporation would be frozen at a manageable level.

2. The high buy-in disincentive to new physicians would be removed.

3. The equity of existing physicians would be recognized through issuance of preferred stock.

4   Additional financing would not be required.

Disadvantages

1. Approval by the Internal Revenue Service was questionable. Under the Internal Revenue Code, the exchange of stock between the two affiliated corporations followed by liquidation of the real estate corporation might not qualify as a tax-free, stock-for-stock exchange for either corporations or shareholders.

2. Under the IRS Code, nonphysician stockholders of the real estate corporation could not be stockholders of a professional corporation. To avoid adverse tax treatment by the IRS, it would therefore be necessary to redeem the shares of the dentists and administrator before a stock-for-stock exchange.

3. Dividends paid to preferred stockholders would not be deductible. Also, the group felt that the dividend treatment of preferred stockholders could create friction between new and old stockholders.

Alternative 2. Recapitalization through Issuance of Promissory Notes

Alternative 2 was similar to Alternative 1 in that stockholders in the real estate corporation would sell all of their shares of stock to the professional services corporation. However, instead of recapitalizing through transfer of stock, the professional services corporation would issue promissory notes. The promissory notes would pay a specified amount of interest to the note holders. As in Alternative 1, the stockholders in the real estate corporation would then buy shares of stock in the professional services corporation at a nominal amount. This would lower the buy-in for new physicians.

Advantages

1. Unfunded growth in the real estate corporation would be frozen at a manageable level.

2. The high buy-in disincentive to new physicians would be removed.

3. The equity of existing physicians would be recognized through issuance of promissory notes.

4. Additional funding would not be required.

5. Interest paid on the notes would be deductible.

Disadvantages

1. Approval by the IRS was questionable because the plan called for transfer of one affiliated corporation to another.

2. Nonphysician stockholders could not be stockholders of a professional service corporation and would have to sell shares back, causing capital gains tax to be due immediately.

3. Different levels of personal equity among existing physicians and new physicians might create friction as time went on.

Alternative 3. Conversion to a General Partnership

Alternative 3 would convert the real estate corporation to a general partnership. The existing shareholders would become general partners.

Advantages

1. This alternative would remove the real estate corporation as a tax paying entity.

2. The new partners would then receive a pass-through of all income and deductions connected with the real estate operation.

3. If the operation continued to produce positive income flow, the income could be used to offset losses the partners might have from other passive activities.

Disadvantages

1. The partners would be jointly and severally liable for all activities connected with the partnership.

2. The liquidation of the real estate corporation would most likely create severe income tax consequences at both the corporate and shareholder levels.

Alternative 4. Acquisition of the Real Estate Corporation

In Alternative 4, the professional service corporation would purchase all of the assets of the real estate corporation. To do this, an MAI appraisal of the building and equipment would have to be performed to establish an arm's-length value of the assets. The professional service corporation would then pay cash for the established value of all of the shares of stock, and the real estate corporation would be liquidated and merged into the professional service corporation.

Advantages

1. The real estate corporation would be liquidated, eliminating the need for a high buy-in.
2. The unfunded growth in the real estate corporation would be capped at the purchase price of the sale.
3. The merger of the two corporations would leave one entity with no strings attached, that is, no preferred stock or interest notes. All physicians would be on a par with each other.
4. All shareholders in the real estate corporation would receive immediate cash disbursement for the value of their shares.

Disadvantages

1. Nonphysician shareholders would no longer have ownership interest in the corporation.
2. It was questionable whether the bank would allow the physicians essentially to leverage the equity of the corporation.
3. There was risk of an IRS challenge of the sale price of one affiliated company to another.
4. Capital gains tax would have to be paid immediately upon the cashing out of the stock.

Alternative Selected

All of the alternatives had their pros and cons. The one constant that kept surfacing in all of the discussions was the desire to have equality in the plan for all shareholders. Alternatives 1 and 2 were variations of the same idea. The fact that neither would require additional financing made them attractive. Ultimately, however, the board rejected them because both required two classes of investment by physicians. Alternative 3, changing to a general partnership, offered many pass-through advantages to the shareholders, but it was rejected because of the adverse tax consequences.

Alternative 4 was selected because it met all of the administrative goals and placed all physicians on an equal investment basis. A plan was presented to the bank, showing the difference in the debt requirement of borrowing the money now to purchase the real estate corporation shares of stock versus the amount that would be necessary in the future under the original plan. The bank agreed with Alternative 4 and approved all of the necessary financing to acquire the real estate corporation. Exhibit 1 is a listing of the documentation needed to complete an acquisition.

Exhibit 1. Documentation Required for Sale of Real Estate Corporation to Professional Service Corporation

---

Real Estate Corporation
- Shareholders' resolution to terminate the stock purchase agreement to permit gifts of stock
- Resolutions authorizing the sale of assets and liquidation of the corporation
- Tender of stock certificates by those making gifts of shares
- New certificates
- Purchase agreement between real estate corporation and professional service corporation for the sale of real estate and other assets
- Deeds for various parcels being conveyed
- Assignment of leases
- Liquidation documentation to be filed with the appropriate state offices

Professional Service Corporation
- Resolutions authorizing the purchase, borrowing of funds, and increase in minimum capital
- Purchase agreement
- Loan documentation (promissory note, mortgage, loan agreement)
- New lease with dental group
- New stock purchase agreement

Closing Statement

The problems facing this group practice under the original plan were: (1) the continual rise in the buy-in requirement of the corporation that was unattractive to physician recruits, (2) the war chest for buying back the shares of retiring physicians was empty, and (3) the growth in the stock of the real estate corporation would be devastating to the corporation in the future. "Biting the bullet" and freezing the rapid growth of the buy-out was an appropriate move for the group practice. Because banks now look not only at the book value of a property, but also at the real market value, the group now regards its buildings as an ongoing expense rather than an appreciating asset. This move put the group in a much better financial position for the future.

Questions for Discussion

1. Why did the author feel the choice of Alternative 4, acquisition of the real estate corporation, would place the group in a better position for the future?

2. If the partners were less concerned about parity of investment, would the choice of alternative have been different?

3. Was the issue of investment by the nonphysicians (the dentists and administrator) a factor in the final decision? If not, why?

4. Why was it so important that the group regard its buildings as an on-going expense rather than an appreciating asset?

CASE 16

Affairs of the Office
When the Physician Becomes Involved

by Anonymous

As the administrator of a ten-physician multispecialty group practice I was involved in the implementation of a three-year business plan in conjunction with the long-range plans of the group. During the development phase of the business plan, the group had decided to upgrade their existing computer systems, including a new computer for third-party billing and a move to computerize and bring all accounting and financial functions in-house. In addition, a move was planned for the independent in-house laboratory to acquire the additional square footage needed to meet the state and federal government's standards for certification. Also, the medical record department needed to increase its size by one-third to accommodate the larger patient base. I had been negotiating with the hospital, which owned the medical building, to obtain space for over two years. Ironically, the space needed for all of the moves became available simultaneously.

Several formal business meetings were initiated with the physicians, managers, and staff to prepare the final plan to accomplish the simultaneous moves. The former computer space was to be renovated to accommodate the laboratory, the former laboratory space was to be renovated to become the new charting area, and new space was being renovated for the billing and financial staff. Under normal circumstances, the above tasks would be formidable; however, we had devised a solid plan and the 40-plus full-time equivalent employees were enthusiastic and prepared for the multiple changes about to take place.

The medical director, elected by the board, was entrusted with the responsibility to interact with the administrator on a daily basis and relate any and all concerns of the physicians during the project. The medical director and I had been working closely for two years organizing the management of the group, and our relationship was professional and interactive. The magnitude of this project necessitated our daily interaction, and during our conversations he began to discuss his family and his personal life. Despite the personal nature of our conversations, I felt empathy for his situation and consoled him by allowing him to vent his sorrow due to his failing marriage. I had no idea of the possible ramifications of these conversations in both a personal and professional sense.

During the renovation of the new billing and financial area, a female employee called me from home. She was hysterical and crying uncontrollably. Since the woman was a long-standing employee and well known to me, I arranged to meet her to attempt to discover the problem at hand. The woman explained that she was having an extramarital affair with the medical director and that she was leaving her husband to be with him. The woman was married to the cousin of the chairman of the board of the primary hospital to which the group admitted its patients. She indicated that, if her husband discovered her infidelity, the group would be in jeopardy because of the political pressure that the chairman of the hospital could impose. I advised the woman to discuss the situation with her family and friends and seek professional help in resolving her immediate crisis.

Upon returning to the office, I was called to the office of the medical director, who was also hysterical and crying uncontrollably. The physician indicated that he was having an affair with the employee but did not know what to do. In addition to being the medical director of the group, he was also the medical director of the hospital. He knew of the connection between the woman and the hospital board and was frightened that, if the affair became public knowledge, it would disgrace him both personally and professionally. Since I had allowed this physician the opportunity to discuss his personal life in the past, I did not prevent him from discussing it at this time. This was poor judgment on my part. I had little perception of how to handle such a personal problem, yet continued to listen and counsel both parties in the hope that the problem would resolve itself. The medical director asked me to keep the problem confidential, and I complied.

Within a week of the telephone call from the woman, the affair became somewhat obvious because the physician and the woman spent an inordinate amount of time behind closed doors. At this point, the physician began spending all of his time between patients in my office. He was asking for advice — he wanted to know what the community would think if knowledge of the affair were to become public, what his wife and children would think, what the other physicians would think, and so forth. I was patient and understanding and offered what support I could, but the physician continued to occupy my time to the point that the business functions necessary to keep the group functioning were being compromised. The contractor needed my approval on his punch list; the computer vendor needed the conversion data prepared and final financial and demographic information presented; the laboratory manager needed my approval on the purchase of additional equipment and for the final laboratory design; equipment and supply vendors were calling and visiting to secure their final bids. Because of my involvement with the medical director and his problems, I was generally unavailable to work with these people during business hours, and changed their meetings to the evening. They were not pleased with these arrangements but complied in order to complete their portion of the project and be paid according to the payment schedule.

I delegated the daily management of the group to the personnel manager, and she undertook the responsibility of assuring professional medical care and smooth patient flow. I delegated the negotiation for some equipment and services to the financial manager. The billing manager assumed the tasks involved with packing and preparing the billing office to move. While the office had always functioned as a team, now the team leader was behind closed doors with the medical director.

I met with the woman to discuss the situation, and it was decided that she would voluntarily leave the employ of the group, in the hope that this change would resolve the physician's day-to-day crisis and return the practice to some semblance of normality.

The physician continued to occupy half of my business time, to the point that my work was being further compromised. I contemplated addressing the situation with the other members of the group. Was it in the best interests of the physician and the group that others be informed? Should the group know the possible ramifications of the particular parties involved? What did the group think was my reason for delaying tasks without obvious cause? Was my reputation as the administrator being damaged by my actions? I grappled with all of the conflicting pieces of the problem and decided to keep the problem confidential.

I spoke to the physician at length and requested that he share his problem with another member of the group and take a leave of absence to make decisions that would affect his personal and professional life. The physician refused this request despite his awareness of possible ramifications if the group were to discover the situation through other sources. In addition, I indicated to him that I was being forced to work 70-plus hours per week because of the time that his personal problems were absorbing from my business day. He was spending all of his free time in my office lamenting his situation, but was unwilling to share the problem with his associates. During this time, various staff members asked me what was wrong. It was apparent that I was not at my usual level of efficiency, but I could not tell them the problem without revealing the situation. They told me later that they thought that the medical director and I were reviewing the work of the contractor and the project as a whole while he was in my office for extended periods.

During the following two months, I began to feel the pressure of the demanding level of work that required my constant attention, and the physician who was controlling much of my time. The frustration of being stifled and unproductive took its toll. I was short-tempered with the staff at a time when they needed my strongest support, and I was beginning to doubt my own efficiency. At this point, both the physician and the woman had sought professional help in coping with their dilemma, but I had not. Although accustomed to dealing in stressful and conflicting business situations on a regular basis, I had never been prepared for the dynamics of this type of personal situation. The turning point occurred during one of the physician's weeping sessions when he was lamenting his desire to leave his family. He needed "a place to think," to clear his thoughts and to come to decisions. With work falling behind and control of the situation lost, I chose the path of least resistance: I gave him the keys to my house. I thought that, by having the physician removed from my office, I would be able to handle the demanding workload that the project demanded.

The physician began using my home to continue his affair. My husband was aware of this arrangement and agreed that it was probably an acceptable short-term solution. He realized the strain that this problem had created in my life and knew the parties involved. He agreed that little harm would arise from allowing the house to be used. After this change, the inordinate amount of my time that the physician occupied was reduced, and I began to regain control of the situation within the office. This turned out to be a brief but problematic reprise.

A month later, the physician shared the details of his affair with the group's president and identified the woman involved. I was greatly relieved and thought that the revelation of these facts to the president would bring some action on the part of the group to address the situation. Again, I was wrong. The president kept the information confidential and did not share it with the board or the other associates within the group.

I decided to meet with the group's president to discuss the situation from both a professional and a personal standpoint. The president indicated that I should do my best and that the group would understand if any delays in the renovations or normal business functions resulted. The president, however, did not inform his associates of the situation. I felt betrayed, frustrated, and personally invaded. I decided to end my personal involvement immediately. I demanded the return of my keys and told the physician to handle his own life and not to interfere in my personal and professional life. The physician was furious and countered that I was feeling overwhelmed by the increased workload and that my reactions were based entirely on this and had nothing to do with his personal problems.

Many questions haunted me during and after this situation. Who was at fault? Should I have been less compassionate and allowed the physician to collapse? Should the president have acted more definitively and set the problem to rest? Did I allow the situation to develop further than it should have? How could the situation have been handled differently?

During the course of these events, I was completely unprepared to handle this type of problem. I made a serious mistake in not soliciting the advice of other administrators and allowing the physician to manipulate me on a personal and professional level. I was in an area of medical group management in which I had no experience, and stumbled through the events as they unfolded.

I acted and reacted on a personal level and allowed my emotions to take control over my business sense.

In retrospect, I see the situation more clearly. My first error in judgment was allowing the physician to discuss his personal life. I should have presented the problem to the board in the beginning stages, but at the time I thought that this would have been a betrayal of personal confidence. In the beginning, when the physician was consuming my business time, I considered forcing him to take his problems to the board. I did not do this, however, because of the pity and empathy I felt toward him. His personal problems clouded my judgment, and I allowed him to continue despite damaging effects.

My second error in judgment was attempting to resolve the situation by removing the physician from the office to my home. I was beset by requests from managers, staff, and vendors and needed business time available. I still did not want to violate the confidential information he shared with me, and made this unsuccessful attempt to resolve the situation by avoiding the issue.

After his revelation of the facts to the president of the group, I thought that the issue would finally be resolved. Despite my long-term relationship with the group and the president, I was dismayed and disappointed by his lack of action. I was counting on someone other than myself, either the medical director or the president, to resolve the problem for me. This was due in part to the increased volume of work required on my part during the renovations, in part to my desire to help the medical director solve his problem, and in part to the confidential nature of the issue. In effect, I did not want to embarrass the medical director in front of his peers with the details of his personal problems and thought that approaching the board would open his personal life to scrutiny. The medical director was performing his medical functions in his usual pattern, and the patients did not suffer because of his personal problems. If his patient care had been compromised, I would have taken the problem directly to the board.

Playing catchup for months of lost time made me angry and resentful of both the medical director and president. I was also angry with the poor judgment I had displayed throughout the entire ordeal. Had I not allowed the physician to share his personal problems, I probably would never have experienced the events that occurred later on. My lack of experience in dealing with this type of situation was a contributing factor, but the fact that I did not seek help from others (e.g. the board, other administrators) indicated my insecurity on the issue, and eventually led to the problems multiplying.

I thrust myself into the workload and completed the new laboratory, record room, and billing office. The new computer system was installed and went live on schedule. The installation of the new system increased the group's gross revenues by 25 percent within three months. The group was thrilled with the success of the project, but I was unhappy and drained. In the end, I offered my resignation to the group. I had succeeded in the project and its goals, but I had failed myself in properly handling the problems with the medical director.

The ultimate irony was the reaction of the physicians, external accountants, and legal counsel when I presented my resignation. The president offered to release the physician from the group and retain me as the administrator. He also informed the group of what had transpired with the physician. Each member of the group spoke with me personally and pleaded that I stay. The president offered a substantial salary and benefit package to me, and three months' paid leave to overcome the trauma of the situation. This outpouring of support came as a great surprise and was somewhat gratifying. Despite this, I could not continue in my capacity with the group. I had not handled the problem properly, and I knew it. I left the group three months later.

I made the mistake of trying to help the medical director with little experience in the area of extramarital affairs and little knowledge of the ramifications of human reactions in such a situation. It is impossible to conjecture what the board would have decided to do had they been informed early on, but it is certain that the problem would have been placed where it belonged, that is, with the board and the physician's peers. It is not the administrator's job to become a marriage counselor or psychotherapist. I assumed both roles in addition to that of administrator. This was certainly an admirable gesture, but one doomed to failure. In addition, as the events unfolded, I did not seek professional advice. I suffered, both personally and professionally, my husband and family suffered, my work suffered, and ultimately I had little left to give to the group and resigned. My desire to help overrode my business sense. I learned the hard way that, when a problem is out of your control, it should stay there, and be placed in the control of those who are in a position to handle it.

Subsequent to my resigning as administrator, the group has continued to flourish both professionally and financially. The physician is separated from his wife, and the woman is divorced from her husband. They are still together. The group hired a competent administrator to replace me and has added three new physicians. Although I have returned on occasion to the former group to present seminars to the physicians and staff on third-party billing and medical management issues, I am now working with another group.

Questions for Discussion

1. Should the administrator have resigned?
2. When should confidences be held as such? What factors might require the overruling of a confidence?
3. What were the personal risks to the administrator in the way she elected to handle the situation?
4. What can you do to prevent such an occurrence from happening?
5. Why did the president elect not to act in a timely fashion?
6. Was the outcome of the problem satisfactory? If not, what else might have been done?

Computer Crash
Living Through Your Worst Nightmare

by Mary E. Ryan

The Sunshine Medical Associates is a ten-physician multispecialty group practice incorporated in 1972. The group began with five physicians and, over a period of 12 years, expanded its size to nine physicians with an active patient base that exceeds 25,000 patients. All of the physicians practice both as primary care physicians and within their specialty. The group members are all board-certified in internal medicine as well as within their specialties, which include oncology, hematology, endocrinology, gastroenterology, infectious diseases, cardiology, family practice, and rheumatology. In addition, the group provides in-house laboratory, radiology, and cardiovascular stress testing.

In 1984, Sue Kelly was hired as the clinic administrator, replacing an office manager who had functioned at a somewhat lower level of responsibility. During the office manager's tenure, the group had successfully moved from the era of ledger cards and typewritten claims to a computerized billing system.

When Ms. Kelly arrived, the group was still functioning without a formal board of directors. Decisions were reached, when possible, after tracking down each physician and requesting an opinion or preference on a suggestion or project. After formal business meetings were arranged, with all of the physicians present, it was decided to create a position for a single physician to act as the physician manager for the group. Ms. Kelly developed a job description and a salary for this position, and the group approved it. They took a vote and chose a physician to serve in this capacity for one calendar year, with subsequent votes to take place annually. The purpose of the physician manager was to act as the intermediary between the individual physicians and the administrator to facilitate the decision-making process on a daily basis.

During Ms. Kelly's conversations with the physician manager, he identified concerns relating to the existing computer system. In particular, the group was not confident that the productivity numbers posted to each physician were correct. Since the division-of-income formula was partially based on the productivity of the individual physicians, Ms. Kelly and the physician manager decided that the first priority was to investigate the system and determine the accuracy of the numbers.

Ms. Kelly initiated the review of the system by identifying each piece of computer hardware within the practice and the work being performed by each staff member on the system. In addition she ran every report available on the system and tracked the remittance advices back through the system to verify the posting of charges and payments to the physician who rendered the service. During this process, Ms. Kelly made some startling discoveries. The system did not, in fact, post the charges and payments to the physician rendering care, but to the physician listed as the patient's primary physician. The last three physicians who joined the group had had significantly lower productivity numbers than the others despite the fact that their schedules were actually overbooked on a daily basis. Upon further investigation, it became apparent that the primary physicians were receiving the credit for the new physicians' productivity.

This finding, unfortunately, was only the beginning of the problems discovered with the system. The practice had a mainframe computer system, which was slow in compiling information and used a reel-to-reel backup system. There were seven computer screens, two printers, and an optical scanner that read the computer card that functioned as an encounter form for each patient. During Ms. Kelly's research, the system went down an average of two to three times per week. The software and hardware vendors could not identify any obstacle that would cause this problem, and the staff were forced to restore the system each time from the backup tapes taken the previous day. Ms. Kelly decided to perform the backup and verification procedures personally to ensure that the stored backup tapes were accurate and could, in fact, be used to restore the system.

Conversations with other practices and computer professionals yielded the suggestion that the system's wiring might be faulty. When Ms. Kelly asked who had wired the system, the staff indicated that the previous office manager had done it herself. Ms. Kelly was astonished by the fact that the system had not been wired by a professional electrician, but apparently, the previous office manager had done the job herself to save money. A licensed electrician familiar with computer wiring was contacted, who then rewired the entire system. Afterward, the system never experienced any downtime, and no restorations were necessary.

In addition to the above problems, the system also had incorrect provider numbers, incorrect location codes, and a variety of other inconsistencies that contributed to a very high rejection rate from the insurance carriers. The staff recoded the entire system, reducing the rejection rate to less than 2 percent within two months. The problem of very slow processing time, however, could not be corrected because of the age of the system.

During this entire process, Ms. Kelly met with the physician manager daily and with the entire group monthly to keep them informed on the project. She recommended that the group modify the division-of-income formula until accurate numbers could be retrieved from the system. After a thorough investigation, she informed the physicians that the present system could not provide them with the financial information they needed. They decided to buy a new system that would perform all of the functions the group required. Ms. Kelly then negotiated with the now-functioning board of directors and obtained budgeting for the purchase of a new computer system during the following fiscal year. The process of obtaining proposals from qualified vendors of medical software and hardware began in the fall of 1990. Ms. Kelly allotted 12 months for the proposal and bidding process and set the proposed live date for the complete conversion for February 1992.

While negotiations were under way for a new system, Ms. Kelly promoted an existing employee to the position of billing manager. The group had hired him the previous year, and he had a thorough working knowledge of the practice's hardware and software. Ms. Kelly worked with him extensively to define specific backup and verification procedures. He was responsible for backing up the system daily and verifying that the backup was accurate. This process required 90 minutes and was performed at the end of each day. The backup tapes were color coded and used sequentially, and each tape was recorded in a backup book for easy identification. In addition, he was responsible for keeping weekly backup tapes in a fireproof safe in his home, storing the daily backup tapes in the on-site fireproof safe. After reviewing his work for a month, Ms. Kelly was satisfied that he was performing the tasks appropriately, and she delegated management of the computer system and billing to him.

In August of 1991, the old computer system went down. There had been no down time since the system had been rewired, and there was no readily identifiable reason why the problem had recurred. The billing manager tried to restore the system, without success, and then requested Ms. Kelly's assistance. While the backup book logged the sequential tapes, the physical tapes were not in proper order. Ms. Kelly attempted several times to restore the system, but was unsuccessful. She then requested that the billing manager go home and retrieve the off-site backup. Surprisingly, he indicated that he did not have an off-site backup. After a lengthy conversation with him in which he offered no explanation for his actions, Ms. Kelly promptly terminated his employment.

The previous May, Ms. Kelly had purged a significant amount of information from the system over a weekend and backed up and verified the tapes. These tapes were at her home, and they were the only tapes that were available. She called the software and hardware vendors and requested that they verify that this one remaining backup was accurate and to make a copy of the tapes. Fortunately, they were able to do this in a timely manner, and the system was restored within two days. However, all of the demographic and financial data for a three-month period was lost, and, with over $3 million in receivables, the implications were overwhelming. Ms. Kelly had met with the physician manager as soon as the restoration problem was discovered, to discuss the ramifications of the data loss. Since the two of them had already discussed the safeguards and procedures Ms. Kelly had put in place to avoid this problem, he agreed that the billing manager was at fault. On a personal level, however, Ms. Kelly admitted that she should have been more careful. She decided she needed to rethink what had gone awry and make changes to ensure that this would never happen again.

The data and media loss coverage on the group's insurance policy was reviewed. Fortunately, the policy had been updated several months before, and coverage for $10,000 was in effect. Ms. Kelly assembled the billing staff for an emergency meeting and created a team to recreate the missing data. They discussed the problems that would occur when payments were received with no charge to which to post them, the problems with patient statements being incorrect during the restoration process, the methodology for restoring the information, and many other factors that would come into play as the restoration process continued. They spoke about the stress of redoing work they had already done and decided to solicit the assistance of the entire organization in the process.

A general staff meeting was held the following day, and Ms. Kelly explained the problem in detail so that everyone would understand. The team would need to review many patient records and laboratory and radiology results, and everyone's cooperation would be needed to complete the task. Two experienced billing staff members were assigned to recreate the missing information, three temporary data entry clerks would assist them in the process, and the two remaining billing members would continue to enter the current information through the optical scanner. Since the scanner was being used for current information, it was not available to recreate data. The team tried, in the evening and on weekends, to put the old computer cards through the scanner, but the cards had been creased when they were filed and no longer worked in the scanner. The only recourse was to recreate the data from the cards and enter the information manually. This process was labor-intensive because the staff had never needed to enter charges manually in the past. The team created a sample computer card, identifying each grid with the proper code, and each biller used the sample to identify the actual charges and payments on the old cards.

The total recreation process took two months and was as accurate as possible under the circumstances. The actual costs incurred were significant and included increased costs for overtime pay and additional temporary employees' pay. The nonmonetary costs were even greater. Ms. Kelly was working 60-hour weeks assisting in the process and assumed responsibility for backup and verification procedures. The billing staff was frazzled and frustrated doing the same work twice. The patients who had changed insurance companies or moved did not have their new information in the system if it was entered during the three- month period. And the physicians were unable to identify referral forms necessary for certain patients. Despite the inaccuracy of the patient billing statements, Ms. Kelly chose to continue mailing the statements to maintain some consistency in the cash flow. The billing staff agreed with this decision, despite the fact that the number of telephone calls would be tremendous. They placed a message on each patient statement, indicating that the group had suffered a loss of data and requesting that the patient call if any information on the statement was incorrect. Most patients did call with updated insurance and demographic information, and when the process was complete the phone calls relating to billing returned to their normal level.

The total cost to recreate the data was a staggering $30,000. The practice collected the $10,000 in data and media loss coverage; however, this left the group with a $20,000 loss, an unacceptable loss by any standard.

Questions for Discussion

1. Can you identify some of the steps that Ms. Kelly might have taken to prevent this crisis?

2. Once the crash occurred, should Ms. Kelly have done anything differently?

3. Should the billing manager have been terminated in such haste? If not, why not?

4. How much control should be vested in one individual — in this case, the administrator?

5. Is there a role for an outside auditor in this situation, and if so, what is that role?

CASE 18

Downsizing at the Dodge Clinic
A Case Study in Three Parts

by Mark Secord

Center City, population 300,000, is located an hour-and-a-half away from a major city. It draws from a wide surrounding rural agricultural region, with a total service-area population of about 500,000. During the 1980s, the population increased by 20 percent, but projections show it is leveling off to about .75 percent growth per year.

Four hospitals serve Center City:

- University Hospital, 350 beds, affiliated with the medical school
- Center City Community Hospital, 330 beds, private, not-for-profit
- St. Elizabeth's Hospital, 400 beds, affiliated with Sisters of Heavenly Bliss
- Plainview Hospital, 250 beds, acquired one year ago by Columbia/HCA

There are two substantial physician group practices. University Associated Physicians consists of 260 members of the medical school faculty and is heavily weighted toward specialists. Dodge Clinic, with 160 physicians, has a mix of about 40 percent primary care physicians and 60 percent specialists. About 65 percent of Dodge's hospital admissions are to Center City Community Hospital.

The health insurance market in Center City is still largely fee-for-service, although mostly discounted through preferred provider organizations. Provider discounting has become increasingly aggressive in the past year. The prepaid capitation market is small at present but growing fast. Within the year, the state plans to implement managed Medicaid in the community. One of the large employers that has a portion of its national workforce in Center City is encouraging its employees to shift to HMO plans. Other employers are show-ing strong interest in this approach. Two years ago, the Dodge Clinic underwent a transition from a partnership form of organization to a not-for-profit founda-tion. It is now governed by a board, two-thirds of whose members are drawn from the community's business and civic leaders. The clinic had considered a merger with Center City Community Hospital, but in the end, the difficult management style of the long-term CEO of the hospital stopped the deal.

Key clinic leaders are Jeffrey Sillman, M.D., president, and John Martin, administrator. Carrying on a tradition established in the clinic's partnership era, the president is elected by the physicians to a three-year term (no consecu-tive terms permitted), and continues to practice medicine on a part-time basis. Dr. Sillman and Mr. Martin jointly chair the management council, a group that meets twice a month and brings together the six physician department chiefs and the clinic's four top administrative staff members. This group makes most major operational decisions.

When the physicians were partners, their income was directly related to the net revenue that they collectively generated. Now they are employees of the corporation with salaries set in advance of the fiscal year, and a portion of their salary is based on the last two years' revenue. The clinic managed to gen-erate a small positive bottom line during the first year of operations in its new corporate form. This year, however, the picture has deteriorated, and through August the clinic shows a year-to-date operating loss of $1.2 million on total revenues of $53.6 million. Part of the clinic's financial difficulties can be traced to an ambitious expansion of primary care, with four new satellite clinics es-tablished in the past two years. A total of 21 physicians were added, most of them in family practice and obstetrics/gynecology.

The clinic is involved in a joint venture with Center City Community Hos-pital, which operates an HMO with about 35,000 members enrolled. The HMO accounts for about 15 percent of the clinic's gross revenues. The clinic is cur-rently receiving a share of the capitation payments that represents 52 percent of the gross charges for this group of the clinic's patients.

Part I. John Martin's Dilemma

John Martin was taking time to do something he rarely did since he took over as administrator of Dodge Clinic — sit at his desk and think. As he reviewed his notes from that morning's management council meeting, he couldn't recall a time during the six months since he had been promoted from chief operating officer to CEO that the physicians were more divided in their opinions — and on such a critical question.

At issue was what to do about the clinic's cost structure. The one thing on which his administrative team and the physician chiefs could agree was that the clinic's costs would have to come down — and pretty fast at that. The big debate was over how fast and by what mechanism those costs ought to be reduced.

They had spent two hours at the council meeting debating the subject with no attempt to reach a decision. But it was time now to decide, especially because the finance committee was meeting in two weeks. The finance committee, especially its hardheaded chairman, Rockney Howard, CEO of ABC Widget Company, would expect clarity and action.

As he reviewed his notes, John Martin could hear the voice of each council member.

Ben Richards, the chief financial officer, usually rather quiet and reserved, was vocal and forceful as he presented the financial picture and set the stage. "We've got to wake up here! We have added costs in this organization like crazy over the past two years, yet doctor productivity has been dropping like a stone! You all know where we stand. At the rate we're losing money, we will see a loss of nearly $3 million by year end, and an even larger loss next year.

"Our management structure and overall operation are sized for the stately business we ran around here a few years ago, when we had a profitable mix of high-end specialists and we got about 75 cents on every dollar of billed charges. Plus, we have added a bunch of management positions associated with our push into primary care satellites and managed care. Now the marketplace is driven by competition based on price. I figure that we need to cut our costs by about 10 percent — and any way you cut it, that is going to translate to about 70 people taken off the payroll. And if we don't get to it soon, we'll be in a deeper hole and we'll have to cut more.

"The way I see it," Mr. Richards continued, "the only way we'll cut this many people out of the place is if we do it pretty much across the board and do it in short order — like within a month. Otherwise, we'll fall into our usual pattern of debating endlessly where cuts can and can't be made, and we'll never actually *do* anything. And the only way we'll get the $7 million in costs is by focusing on head count. True, there are some nonstaff costs we should attack, but we've already cut them pretty hard. And we can't leave the physicians untouched either. Nearly half of our operating expenses are physician salaries. Personally, I would favor using this opportunity to terminate some of the marginal producers, and not penalizing the doctors who are really giving it their all. But, if that pill is too tough to swallow, then we need to make some salary and benefit cuts."

Gareth Williams, chief of surgery, cautioned against cuts in physician income. "Laying off doctors is simply out of the question, and pay cuts aren't much better. We've got to recognize how sensitive the physicians are to the loss of their status as partners. Besides, our doctor salaries aren't out of line with those of comparable clinics, let alone the market in the local community. How can we even think about penalizing the high producers for decisions to hire a slew of family practitioners and OB/GYNs that they went along with reluctantly?"

Dr. Williams added, "I do agree with Ben that we've got to do something about the bloated management structure around here though. Why we need all of these layers between my office assistant and the CEO is beyond me. We can probably top General Motors in that department. Also, we've got way too many nurses around here these days. Why does every obstetrician and every cardiologist need a personal RN?"

Rick Myers, associate administrator, was predictably true to his deeply held personal belief in the total quality philosophy. "If we resort to slash and burn tactics like Ben is suggesting, we'll be throwing out four years' worth of investment in our CQI effort. We're just beginning to build an atmosphere of safety here that allows people to come out of the woodwork with their ideas for improving processes. Laying people off would put so much fear into the ranks that we'd be shooting ourselves in the foot. What would we say to the 20 CQI teams working on the quality council's priority areas? And we've got probably another 40 informal teams under way too.

"We know that CQI can produce cost savings — the teams that have worked on radiology processes have demonstrated that with the reduction in FTEs that resulted from improving scheduling, patient flow, and room turnover. What we need is time for our investment in CQI to pay off. We may see our bottom line in the red for a year or two while we improve our work processes. But let's sell the finance committee on the idea that these short-term losses are an investment. The important thing is that we engage the whole staff in working our way out of the problem, and that we be able to show continual, measurable progress toward improving the value of our services."

Jim Pederson, chief of medicine, had focused on incentives — as he always did in a discussion like this. "When we gave up the partnership, we lost the doctors' attention to the clinic's financial position. It used to be that Ben would get a flurry of calls prior to the quarterly partnership distributions, to see how the numbers were shaping up. Now, with everyone on a salary, we're insulated from it. Frankly, I think everyone in this place needs to feel an element of financial risk — physicians and other staff alike. If you solve this problem, a lot of other things will fall into place."

Dr. Pederson went on to say, "I differ from Gareth in that I don't think we can leave the physicians untouched in all of this. If employees feel that they are making all the sacrifices just to keep doctor income where it is today, morale will suffer. We'll lose some of our best people."

Ginger Waxman, associate administrator for patient care services, surprised the group with her view of the situation. "I agree with Ben that we need to take more decisive action on head count. We've got too many bodies around this place — too much management structure, too many fiefdoms. But I also think we need outside help to move the change process fast enough — we'll never do it on our own. Nursing is a good example. We've got to break the habit of each physician having a dedicated nurse or office assistant. It's a concept that went out at most other clinics years ago, but we've got a bunch of people — nurses and physicians alike — who bury the idea every time we advance it.

"We need to do what St. Elizabeth's did with its primary care clinic group, and pull in reengineering consultants to help us do the job. Part of what they do is hold everybody's feet to the fire. They'll also bring lots of benchmarking data on other clinics they've worked in, and a clear process to get the job done. It's sort of like CQI in overdrive. It may cost us about $1 million in fees, but the savings will be many more times that."

Pat Abramson, the chief of service departments (laboratory and radiology), took still a different view. "I don't like the idea of using the outside consultants. The truth is that all of us know already where there is fat in the organization. Ginger, you know what you need to do in terms of changing the ratios and staffing mix in nursing. We know that there are redundancies and weak performers in our management structure. Look at the fact that we've got separate managers for engineering, facilities planning, and general services for example. There are some sacred cows with the physician staff — like the two positions in the library that are so important to Dr. Jones. The point is that we already know where there is probably 5 percent in excess cost. All we've lacked is the mandate and the will to get the job done.

"I think we need to give ourselves the discipline of a tight timetable — two months should do — and plan for layoffs as a part of the overall process. We've already got the freeze on hiring in effect, so employees won't be terribly surprised. Sure, it will take people a while to recover from the pain of losing people, but in the long run I think it will make our CQI effort even stronger. We can weed out some of the managers that will probably never be on board with the basic philosophy of CQI, and besides, I think a dose of fear would do the organization good. It's not as if we're dreaming this up in this room — it's our customers who are demanding that we give them better value for their health care dollar."

Tom March, the vice president for human resources, cautioned against the layoffs. "I've been there before folks. In my job at Crown Manufacturing, I saw the impact that a big layoff can have. The morale was still in the tank when I left, and that was a year-and-a-half after the layoff. And it's not as inexpensive in the short term as you think. Severance, unemployment compensation, and outplacement costs really add up.

"How can we say things like 'Join the Caring Team' in our ads in the paper, and hand out copies of our quality vision statement that talk about being 'All One Team,' and having a 'supportive culture where employee input is critical,' and then turn around and fire a bunch of people? It doesn't make sense. What makes sense is putting some resources into that staff training and development center idea that has been knocked out of the budget in the last two years. That way, we could retool people so we can move them into the areas of the organization where there are jobs, like the primary care group."

Neither John Martin nor the president, Jeff Sillman, had taken a stand in the management council meeting, preferring to hear the thoughts of the other members of the group. Now it was time for taking a stand, and Mr. Martin wanted to go into his meeting with Dr. Sillman the next morning with his own views crystallized.

As John Martin pondered the discussion, he found himself coming back to the finance committee. He knew what Rockney Howard would do if he were in his shoes, because he had done it at ABC Widget Company. He would lay off 70 people without a second thought. But there would be other members of the committee more in tune with the total quality management philosophy, willing to give more time and accomplish the change more gradually.

Mr. Martin added up the pros and cons of the various approaches. He decided that he would recommend to Jeff Sillman and the management council laying out several alternative approaches for the finance committee, letting them know that management had considered a range of possible strategies for dealing with the problem. But he would recommend an intermediate course, and plan for a modest-sized layoff — maybe 40 to 50 people — taking advantage of some of those places to cut costs that Dr. Abramson had talked about. But beyond this immediate cost-reduction effort, Mr. Martin would recommend the clinic emphasize process improvement as a critical strategy, with most of the labor savings, he hoped, coming out of attrition over the next two years or so.

Questions for Discussion

1. What do you think of John Martin's recommendation? What are the major advantages and disadvantages of his recommendation?

2. Are there other alternatives that the administrative group may not have talked about that should be considered?

3. What are some of the steps that Mr. Martin and the administrative staff will need to take to keep the hospital's CQI effort moving forward, assuming that the clinic proceeds with layoffs?

Part II. Downsizing Decisions (Three Weeks Later)

Ginger Waxman, the associate administrator for patient care services at Dodge Clinic, was agonizing over the decisions she had to make. The clinic administrative staff had agreed on a target of removing approximately 25 percent of the organization's management positions. There was no question that the clinic's management staff had become bloated over the years. But now came the tough part: which people would be terminated?

Actually, some of the decisions had been easier to make than Ms. Waxman had thought. After the administrative team had examined the problem and developed the overall framework for management reductions, Ms. Waxman had taken the issue to her group of direct reports, calling a special meeting to fill them in on the plan that had been developed to that point. Her philosophy was that it would be best to be open and honest with her managers, even though it was clear that some in the room would be losing their jobs. The meeting didn't last long; it wasn't the kind of subject matter that could be discussed as a group. She delivered the sober message, there was a bit of gallows humor from the group, and they disbanded. But Ms. Waxman had given the message that she really was open to ideas from the group. There were some good ones. In fact, remarkably, one of the managers had stopped by Ginger Waxman's office the following day to tell her that he thought his own position could be consolidated with one in the neighboring section, and he volunteered to be the one to leave the organization.

But now Ms. Waxman was down to the really hard choices. One of the decisions that she was losing sleep over related to the management of the endocrinology section. On paper, without considering the people that occupied the positions, the decision was simple. The position of diabetes center manager would have to be eliminated and the responsibilities incorporated with those of the manager of the endocrinology section. The clinic couldn't afford to keep both managers.

About three years ago, management of the diabetes training program, a well-established program that trains diabetic patients in the proper management of their disease, was the responsibility of Susan Wellworth, the endocrinology section manager. But at that time, the endocrinologists had been approached by executives from U.S. Diacare, an aggressive for-profit chain of diabetes centers whose modus operandi was to form a joint venture with a group of doctors and a local hospital and install a set of management, marketing, and clinical procedures. What attracted the Dodge Clinic endocrinologists was the prospect of a dramatic increase in market share, which, U. S. Diacare assured would come when the chain's expertise was brought to bear. Neither Ginger Waxman, John Martin, nor the administrator of Center City Hospital was impressed when they reviewed the full U. S. Diacare business plan. True, other medical groups and hospitals had done quite well with the company's program, but it amounted to a big share of the profits leaving the local providers. Why not beef up the program themselves, they reasoned?

This led to the hiring of Fritz Weisman, and it had proven to be a great decision. An affable and smart young manager, Mr. Weisman had done an outstanding job as manager for diabetes care. He had doubled the program's patient volume by coordinating a major marketing effort and initiating a series of innovative program improvements. He rebuilt the diabetes center staff, dealing with some of the long-standing interpersonal conflicts that had plagued the program for years.

It turned out that Mr. Weisman was one of the clinic's early converts to CQI, and senior leadership often used his department as an example of what CQI in daily work life should look like. The ten-member staff had all been taught CQI methods and tools. Each of them was involved in several improvement-team projects, and most could address how they applied the plan/do/check/act cycle in their own work on a regular basis. Customer satisfaction and patient outcomes were measured routinely, and control charts and histograms papered the walls in the staff area of the diabetes center. Most of all, anyone who walked in the door of the center could instantly sense the atmosphere of staff involvement and commitment to the program. To the staff, Mr. Weisman was a coach, a teacher, a leader, but he wasn't a "boss" in the traditional sense.

Because of his knowledge about CQI and his credibility with other managers in the clinic, Mr. Weisman had been pulled into a broader role in the organization's CQI effort. He received special training as a facilitator and served in this capacity for several multidisciplinary process-improvement teams. He was part of the in-house faculty group that taught other managers and physicians CQI methods and tools in the clinic's training course.

But on the organization chart, it was apparent that Mr. Weisman's position would have to go, and that his management duties for the diabetes center should be given back to Susan Wellworth. There was no question, given the current smooth-running operation in the diabetes program, that Susan Wellworth could manage both operations. Moreover, she had been with the organization for nearly 20 years, and was well-liked and respected by the physicians and other staff as a solid, competent nurse manager.

So there was no doubt in Ginger Waxman's mind that Fritz Weisman's position would need to be eliminated as a part of the overall clinic reorganization. In fact, in order to make the many difficult and painful decisions elsewhere in the organization "stick," this change would have to be made. Still, she agonized about this decision. It was hard to terminate someone who showed so much promise and who was such a visible person in the clinic's CQI effort.

The other person about whom Ms. Waxman worried was the manager of the clinic's endoscopy suite, Judy Smith. As in the situation in the endocrinology/diabetes center, the consolidation of Judy Smith's unit with other surgical and special procedures units made lots of sense from the standpoint of organizational function and efficiency. In fact, the clinic administrators had attempted to carry out this consolidation several years ago, but the powerful physician head of the gastroenterology section had put his foot down and the idea hadn't gone anywhere. Besides, Judy Smith wasn't a standout manager. She was competent working with her small staff in the endoscopy area but did not have the skills to take on a much larger, more complex job assignment.

The problem was that Judy Smith meant so much more to the clinic than anything written in her job description. She had just received her 25-year pin from the clinic. She was, in a real sense, one of the people who kept the nonphysician staff glued together. She was totally dedicated to the organization and a patient advocate. When there was a party to be organized or a sad event to be dealt with, Judy Smith was there to get people organized, to pull them together. She had a wonderful sense of humor and was gifted at helping the clinic laugh at itself when that was needed.

So, while Ginger Waxman had a list of 11 people whose positions were targeted for elimination, she was really stewing about certain ones. The common element was that these were people whose importance to the organization had less to do with their specific jobs than it did with their broader effect on the Dodge Clinic.

Questions for Discussion

1. Imagine that you are John Martin and that Ginger Waxman has just come to see you, seeking your input and advice on these two decisions. What would you tell her?

2. Assuming that the clinic's leadership proceeds with laying off these two key people and others who have made substantial contributions to the organization during their tenure, what steps should they take to keep the clinic's organizational culture as healthy as possible?

Part III. The Aftermath of Downsizing (Eight Months Later)

John Martin was on an airplane on his way to join his wife and family, who were already on vacation. It was his first vacation in a long time. It had been eight exhausting months since November 2, the day last year that the clinic staff came to call Black Thursday. The date marked the first layoffs in the clinic's history, with 32 people, about half of them managers, being told they had to leave the organization. (A total of 54 positions were eliminated, but some positions were already vacant, and a few people were able to shift to other positions.)

The time leading up to the layoffs and the several months following were the most traumatic of his management career, he reflected. It was gut-wrenching to know that you were responsible for making the decisions that so deeply affected the lives of those involved, both those who had been asked to leave the organization and those who stayed. While the decisions about which positions to eliminate were made in a reasoned way, and the process was conducted in the most humane way possible, the memory of that time left a pit in his stomach.

With a few exceptions, the people who were forced to leave were doing extremely well. Many had found excellent new jobs; most reported that it was a move that they were glad to have made — once they had gotten over the initial shock. Apart from a few of the long-tenured managers who were bitter and angry over the decisions, most seemed to accept the reasoning for the decisions and appreciated the outplacement services made available to them and the reasonably generous severance packages they received.

One thing Mr. Martin would have done differently would have been to hold more formal "goodbye" sessions for those leaving. He had not done this, and the result was that people felt that members of the Dodge Clinic family had simply disappeared.

What had been a surprise to him was the extent of the "survivor's sickness" that prevailed among so many of the clinic staff — physicians, managers, everybody. There were really three categories of staff reactions. For months following Black Thursday, a small minority of staff were downright depressed, seemingly consumed by their feelings of grief and unable to function. Another group were on the opposite end of the spectrum. Soon after the downsizing, they were energized, excited about some of the opportunities for change and looking at old problems in a new light. Most managers and staff were in between, vacillating between the two sets of emotional reactions. The physician group showed some of this behavior as well: one day up, the next down.

In addition, people were incredibly stressed by the increase in workload in the downsized organization. Starting with administration, where one of the positions was eliminated, and throughout the management organization, managers really had their hands full. Even though they were encouraged to find ways to reorganize their work, it was hard to make this a reality and many were putting in extralong hours.

What made matters more difficult was that the financial situation didn't immediately improve. The clinic had ended the year about $2 million behind budget, and the need for another round of serious cost cutting — if not more layoffs — was approaching. Everyone sensed this.

The physicians were extremely restless. While a decision had been made not to include some of the low-producing physicians among those to be laid off last November, for fear of the effect that this might have on the remainder of the group, the sense was widespread that "the other shoe" was going to drop sometime soon. Even some of the clinic's solid producers among the physician staff were given to wondering about their impending doom.

While some of the perks and benefits offered to physicians were trimmed in the expense-reduction effort, there was a feeling of resentment among many of the managers and nonphysician staff that the doctors had escaped the same level of reduction that others had borne.

CQI efforts at Dodge Clinic since November had had mixed results. Several of the staff and managers who were facilitators and pivotal members of process-improvement teams had lost their jobs. Many of the teams and projects under way had lost ground in the face of anxiety about job loss. But there was an unmistakable seriousness and energy behind other improvement efforts. One of the managers put it this way, "I never want to have to go through downsizing again if I can help it, and CQI is the right way to get rid of waste around here."

In short, even eight months later there were lingering effects from the downsizing. John Martin needed a vacation from it all and was finally going to get one — at least for the next ten days. But when he returned from vacation, he needed to move forward and continue the process of healing the clinic's culture.

Questions for Discussion

1. Can you think of some things that Dodge Clinic might have done at the time of the layoffs to ease their impact on the organization?

2. What were the advantages and disadvantages of not laying off low-producing physicians as a part of the downsizing?

3. What steps should the clinic leadership now undertake to heal the wounds of the downsizing and help rebuild staff morale?

4. What are some steps that can be taken to keep the clinic's CQI effort moving forward in the wake of the downsizing?

Mergers and Acquisitions

Hospital Consolidation
Optimal Strategy for a Two-Hospital Town

by Bruce Deal and John F. Tiscornia

John Tortini and the rest of the consulting team sat around the large conference table and reviewed the outline of their final report, which was due in two weeks. The consultants had been asked by the boards of directors of the only two hospitals in Gorsich, Wyoming to study the best possible ways in which the hospitals might work together to meet the health care needs of the community, and Mr. Tortini wanted to be sure everyone was in agreement before the team made its recommendations.

From past experience, Mr. Tortini knew that collaboration between two competing hospitals is never easy, and that the team's report was likely to be attacked by those who opposed the conclusions. Consequently, he wanted to be sure they had covered all of the relevant issues and considered the potential sources of opposition prior to submitting the report.

At the beginning of the meeting, Mr. Tortini asked the various team members to review the findings of the previous eight weeks of on-site work in Gorsich. Bill Dean began the discussion with a review of the financial situation and environment within which the hospitals operate.

Environment and Financial Factors

Holy Family Hospital and Gorsich General Hospital are the only two acute care hospitals in a county of 80,000 people. They also serve as regional referral hospitals for a much larger secondary service area that includes another 90,000 people and 14 small hospitals. Because of the predominant rural nature of the state, patients often travel great distances to receive care. The total service area for the hospitals covers an area approximately five times the size of the state of New Jersey.

The hospitals are located three miles apart in the city of Gorsich, and they are both full-service acute care hospitals, offering nearly a full range of secondary services and some tertiary services. While some services, such as open-heart surgery, are provided only at one hospital, the majority of services are duplicated at the two facilities. Historical market share analysis shows that Gorsich General had an overall 60 percent market share in the county, with Holy Family holding steady at an approximately 40 percent market share. Generally, the community has been very loyal to the two hospitals, which together account for nearly 97 percent of the inpatient volume of the county.

Both hospitals have a long history in the region. Holy Family Hospital was founded by the Sisters of Health Care in the late 1800s and is currently part of Healthcare Services, a loosely affiliated system that includes 14 Catholic hospitals throughout the region. Gorsich General has been in the community for nearly as long as Holy Family, although it is no longer affiliated with its Lutheran founders and now serves as an independent, not-for-profit institution.

The region surrounding Gorsich has generally seen a slowly declining population, especially after the closure of one of the largest employers — a mining smelter — in the middle 1980s. Although unemployment has declined in recent years, many local business leaders are concerned about the long-term economy. The largest employer in the region is Zebra Air Force Base, which is in danger of being downsized or closed due to reductions in defense spending. Many other local employers have also experienced layoffs or downsizing, whereas the hospitals are two of the largest and most stable employers in the region, together accounting for nearly 1,800 full-time equivalent employees.

On the positive side, educational attainment in the region is higher than the national average, although local officials are frustrated that the available jobs often do not take advantage of the well-educated workforce. Many local jobs pay only slightly over minimum wage; many families struggle to get by from paycheck to paycheck. A review of the census data indicates that over 60 percent of the population has an annual household income of less than $30,000 per year, compared to 50 percent of the national population. The weak economy also manifests itself in the health care arena: 15 percent of the population is without health insurance, although 85 percent of the adults in this group are employed in low-wage jobs. While access to emergency care is available from the hospitals and local physicians without regard to ability to pay, lack of insurance is a major barrier to needed preventive and general health care services.

Public health officials are concerned about a number of other local health issues. These include higher-than-average rates of heart disease and cancer, high rates of death and disability from work-related injuries, high adolescent suicide rates, higher out-of-wedlock birthrates than other similar communities in the state, and high rates of alcohol and smokeless tobacco use among the youth of the region. Many of these concerns are not only local issues, but also occur throughout the state, due in part to the weak state-level support for public health efforts.

Mr. Dean proceeded with his review of the environment by detailing some hospital operating statistics the team had compiled during their study. As in nearly all communities around the country, Gorsich has seen a dramatic decrease in the inpatient utilization of hospitals in recent years. As lengths of stay have declined and many services have switched to outpatient settings, the combined acute care average daily census (ADC) of the two hospitals has dropped from nearly 300 in 1983 to just over 150 in 1993. Moreover, these changes occurred in the absence of managed care, which is still nearly nonexistent in the region. The consulting team has estimated that an additional 25 percent decline in the ADC could result when managed care pressures do arrive.

The substantial overcapacity resulting from these changes was one of the key drivers behind the hospitals exploring collaborative activities after decades of competition; the decline in patient volumes made it difficult for both hospitals to maintain staff proficiency and efficient staffing levels in many areas. For example, both hospitals have pediatric units, with reported ADC levels of six patients at one hospital and three patients at the other. Despite these low volumes, physicians working at both hospitals expect nursing and ancillary staff to be fully proficient in nearly all areas.

While inpatient hospital volumes have been decreasing, hospital costs have been increasing substantially. Over the ten-year period ending in 1993, the combined hospital operating costs in Gorsich increased by 115 percent (versus 45 percent for the general inflation level and 100 percent for the national health care inflation level). Indeed, over the previous four years, average price increases by the hospitals were between 8 percent and 9 percent, while per capita income for the state grew by only 4 percent to 5 percent per year. Business leaders interviewed during the project indicated their ability to absorb additional health care cost increases was nearly exhausted, and that some way of controlling local health care costs needed to be found.

Mr. Dean also covered the historical and anticipated future financial results for the hospitals. Both hospitals are currently financially healthy and profitable, although they have both had to resort to staff layoffs and salary freezes during the past two years to avoid operating losses. Neither hospital has a tremendous amount of debt outstanding, and neither is planning a large debt-financed project in the near future. Although neither hospital is an A-rated credit risk in all areas, both are in generally good financial shape at the present time.

A look into the future provided by the consulting team, however, indicates things may get much more difficult financially for the hospitals. As commercial payers begin demanding discounts on hospital charges, patient lengths of stay continue to decline, and government payers continue to cut back, the hospitals are likely to face significant financial losses within the next five years. In essence, they will be fighting over a shrinking patient population, while not being able to make significant reductions in their expenses. While some individuals and physicians at the hospital do not agree with this assessment, the majority of management personnel at both institutions see these trends occurring throughout the country and feel the trends will likely come to Gorsich within the next few years.

Bill Dean concluded his presentation to his colleagues with a discussion of the estimates of cost savings associated with collaborative efforts. For purposes of making estimates, the team developed four alternative scenarios:

- The first alternative is to do nothing and maintain the status quo, which of course would not yield any cost savings.
- The second alternative is to develop a series of joint ventures for some services, such as selected administrative or clinical services, in order to reduce costs through economies of scale. The team had estimated this alternative would save approximately $1.2 million per year in operating costs, which is roughly 1 percent of the annual combined operating budget. In addition, this alternative would allow the hospitals to avoid $3.5 million in duplicated capital spending over the next five years.
- The third alternative is to consolidate the hospitals into a single organization, but maintain selected inpatient services at both facilities. This would likely save approximately $5.8 million per year in operating costs, and $11.5 million over the next five years in capital costs.
- The fourth alternative is to consolidate the hospitals and concentrate all inpatient services at one campus and put many nonacute and ambulatory services at the alternative location. Because of the concentration of acute care services and the resulting economies of scale, this alternative yields the greatest savings — $8 million per year in operating costs, and $14.5 million over the next five years in capital costs.

After Mr. Dean had completed his presentation, Mr. Tortini asked Dustin Robb to review what the team had found during the interview phase of the project. Mr. Robb began with an overview of the process the team had used for its interviews.

Interview Findings

The team spent the first few weeks of the project conducting over 200 interviews with local physicians, hospital personnel, community leaders, public health officials, and payers. The interviews lasted approximately one hour each, and the consultants used a confidential questionnaire to ensure the consistency of the questions being asked.

The team generally found a high degree of support for hospital collaboration from those in Gorsich, although there was dissension within some groups with regard to the desirability of collaboration. One question asked respondents what degree of collaboration they would favor, ranging from 1 being "no collaboration" to 10 being "complete consolidation." The results of this question are shown in Table 1.

Table 1. What Degree of Collaboration Would You Support?					

(1 = Status Quo, 10 = Complete Consolidation)

	1–2	*3–4*	*5–6*	*7–10*	*Responses*
Community and Other	0%	3%	25%	72%	39
Independent MDs	17%	11%	19%	53%	36
Clinic MDs	0%	7%	29%	64%	14
Board Members	0%	0%	15%	85%	19
Mgmt. and Employees	3%	10%	26%	61%	39
Totals	5%	7%	23%	65%	147

As Dustin Robb reviewed these findings with the consulting team, he explained the differences in opinion between the independent physicians and the clinic physicians. The medical community in Gorsich is split fairly evenly between one large multispecialty clinic of about 60 physicians — Gorsich Clinic — and the remaining physicians, organized as independent solo practices and small groups. Gorsich Clinic recently moved into a new building adjacent to Gorsich General and has been fairly aggressively adding new physicians and recruiting existing independent physicians. The remaining independent physicians are largely clustered in hospital-owned medical office buildings around Holy Family Hospital, whose administrator sees part of the hospital's role as a haven for independent physicians who do not want to join Gorsich Clinic.

As the interview results indicate, the Gorsich Clinic physicians are generally supportive of a consolidation of the hospitals. The independent physicians are much less enthusiastic, with a small core group strongly opposed to any collaboration. Mr. Robb speculated that the reluctance of the independent physicians comes from several sources. First, the rural, frontier nature of the region attracts very independent physicians who strongly believe in competition and the survival of the fittest and are opposed to anything they perceive to be reducing competition. Second, a small group of independent physicians are very strongly opposed to either state or national health reform, and these physicians may believe anything that changes the status quo is undesirable. Finally, Mr. Robb felt the independent physicians are fearful that any collaboration between the hospitals would result in a stronger role for Gorsich Clinic within the medical community, possibly to the detriment of the independent physicians.

Apart from the physicians, there appears to be fairly strong support in the community for collaboration or even consolidation. Many local leaders expressed frustration during the interviews at the competition between the hospitals and felt it had only led to unnecessary duplication and additional expense for the community. Many cited the presence of a magnetic resonance imaging unit at each hospital in Gorsich, both of which units are substantially underutilized, as an example of this. Community leaders wondered aloud during the interviews why the hospitals couldn't work together to prevent the unnecessary and expensive duplication.

Finally, Mr. Robb reviewed some of the issues that had surfaced in the interviews that might be barriers to collaboration. A number of people affiliated with both hospitals cited a difference in organizational culture as a potential barrier. The general perception was that Holy Family Hospital is the smaller, more caring, more mission-oriented hospital, while Gorsich General is more "high-tech" and operated more "like a business." Some employees felt it would be difficult to integrate these two cultures in collaborative ventures. In addition, some Holy Family physicians and employees were very concerned that collaborative efforts would lead to a reduction in the Catholic presence or an abandonment of Catholic standards for women's health, which was for some a very strong reason for their affiliation with Holy Family.

After listening to these presentations, John Tortini decided to spend a few minutes reviewing for the team what he had learned about the personalities of the key players involved in the decision-making process. As team leader, Mr. Tortini had spent a lot of time with the CEOs and the board chairs for both hospitals, and his years of experience had given him some insight into players' possible reactions to various recommendations. While it was important to consider the various constituencies, ultimately it would be the boards who would make the final decision.

Key Decision Makers

Mr. Tortini began his review with Scott McDougal and Terry Conrad, who chaired the boards of Gorsich General and Holy Family Hospitals, respectively. Mr. McDougal is the president of the chamber of commerce and is very well known and well respected around the town. Mr. Conrad is the manager of a large construction company and has been active in community affairs for many years. The two men have had a long-standing relationship. Mr. McDougal also had the distinction of being the first lay chair of the Holy Family board, which now draws a majority of its members from the laity. Both Mr. McDougal and Mr. Conrad seem very committed to the process, and Mr. Tortini felt they would seriously consider any recommendation, including a recommendation to consolidate the two organizations into a single entity.

Mr. Tortini then discussed the two CEOs with the team. Jeff Williams, the CEO of Gorsich General, is the younger and more aggressive of the two. Although the exact origin of the idea of a collaboration study was somewhat unclear, it was Mr. Williams who took the initiative to contact John Tortini, and it was clear that Mr. Williams saw himself as the CEO of the new organization if a consolidation did occur. Mr. Williams is in his middle forties and has been

CEO of Gorsich General for approximately six years. In an earlier phase of his career, he had been on the administrative staff at Holy Family Hospital, and thus had a greater degree of familiarity with the workings of the rival hospital than would ordinarily be the case. Mr. Williams is seen by many at both hospitals as being very bright, but possessing a tendency to change things without considering all of the implications of his decisions.

Bob Grambinski, the CEO of Holy Family Hospital, is nearly the complete opposite of Jeff Williams. Mr. Grambinski is 63 and is planning to retire within the next couple of years. He has been at Holy Family for approximately ten years and is seen as a traditional administrator who views himself as the spokesperson for the hospital and the protector of the employees. He leaves the details of running the hospital to his group of three vice presidents, who are each given a great deal of autonomy. Mr. Grambinski is not felt by the employees or the board members to be a strong innovator, but he is universally liked and respected.

John Tortini then discussed the nature of the relationship between the two CEOs. Because of their very different personalities and management styles, they do not work well together. Mr. Grambinski gets frustrated very quickly with Mr. William's "micro-managing" and does not like to be in long meetings with him. Although Mr. Grambinski has not come right out and said so, he does not seem entirely comfortable with Mr. Williams being the CEO if a consolidation occurs. In fact, while Mr. Grambinski is generally in favor of collaboration, he has expressed reservations about moving too quickly toward that goal. He has suggested it may make sense for the hospitals to spend some time "getting to know each other," in collaborative ventures, before undertaking a consolidation.

Mr. Tortini finished his review by discussing Miranda Maddern, the CEO of Healthcare Services, the parent organization of Holy Family Hospital. Healthcare Services is a fairly loose affiliation of the local Sisters of Health Care Catholic hospitals in the region, with Ms. Maddern and a few others being the only employees of the corporate office. Ms. Maddern has been CEO of Healthcare Services for only one year, having formerly been one of the founders of a small health care consulting firm. She is a dynamic and, at times, opinionated manager who understands the problems of overcapacity and other issues, and generally looks favorably upon collaborative efforts. She seems to see her role as both ensuring that Holy Hospital actively participates in the process, and positioning Healthcare Services to have some role in whatever entity evolves from the discussions. She will also serve as liaison with the Sisters of Health Care, who will ultimately have to approve any changes at Holy Family Hospital.

Other Issues

After a short break for lunch, John Tortini reconvened the meeting and opened the floor for discussion. Bill Dean began by saying that, while he generally supported a consolidation of the organizations based on the data, he felt the opportunity to be constrained by the physical facilities of each hospital. Gorsich General is the larger of the two hospitals, although it is still slightly too small to accommodate the entire current inpatient and outpatient volumes of both hospitals. It is also nearly 30 years old and in need of some substantial renovations, including asbestos removal. Unfortunately, renovations alone may not be enough. The floor plan is not particularly efficient and, due to the presence of many hallways and small rooms, the hospital has the feel of a "rabbit warren," as one of the other team members described it.

Holy Family Hospital, on the other hand, was constructed on a new location in the 1970s and has recently added a new emergency room and rehabilitation wing. The facility is in good shape but is significantly too small to accommodate the entire volume of both hospitals. To locate all services on the Holy Family campus would require a major capital campaign involving tens of millions of dollars, which does not seem likely in the near future. While data from other communities would indicate that the greatest savings come from a consolidation onto one campus, this does not seem possible in this situation. And, while the savings from collaborative efforts may be substantial, they will not be as great as those under full consolidation.

Dustin Robb then brought up the likely objections to any recommendation for collaboration or consolidation. First, the independent, more conservative physicians were likely to object on the grounds that any reduction in competition is undesirable. From the physicians' standpoint, many of them have been able to exploit the two hospitals for equipment and other favors, and a consolidation would eliminate this opportunity.

In addition to the independent physicians, some opposition to collaboration would be likely from employees of the two hospitals. While everyone is in favor of reducing health care costs, cost reductions ultimately translate into reductions in jobs and possibly layoffs. There are not many opportunities in Gorsich for other good jobs, so employees concerned about losing their jobs may find it difficult to support collaborative efforts. Finally, Mr. Robb continued, religious issues may surface and create opposition to collaboration. Anti-abortion forces had picketed Gorsich General in the past, and they could create problems throughout the discussions by focusing attention on the abortion and sterilization issues.

John Tortini wrapped up the discussion with a review of the antitrust issues. If the hospitals did decide to collaborate to the point of consolidating operations, the move would require approval from either the Justice Department or the Federal Trade Commission. Both of these organizations have gone on record recently opposing consolidations in situations similar to that in Gorsich. Their position is that consolidations that create monopolies result in higher prices and lower quality than would otherwise be the case. While this is not necessarily the position of many experts with regard to the market for health care services, a consolidation would nonetheless likely involve a fight with the federal antitrust agencies. If very strong community support for a consolidation were forthcoming, then the fight might be won without going to court, but this is considered an unknown at this point.

With the afternoon drawing to a close, and the pros and cons having been presented, Mr. Tortini decided it was time for a decision. He began by going around the room asking each member of the team for a recommendation.

Questions for Discussion

1. What would your recommendation be? Why?

2. If you would recommend a consolidation, how would you recommend the hospitals proceed?

3. How would you propose the consultants communicate their recommendations (e.g., closed meetings versus public meetings, press coverage versus no press coverage)?

4. What strategy should the hospitals and their consultants adopt with regard to potential opposition groups?

CASE 20

Merger or Independence
Small Group Decision — Large Group Impact

by D. Cheryl Erins

The primary care practice, not unlike other small group private practices, was faced with many challenges, including the inability to attract and retain qualified physicians, spiraling overhead costs, encroachment of insurance company and hospital-based primary care practices, and decreasing enjoyment of lifestyles on the part of the group's established physicians. As a result, it became necessary to develop a proactive process, evaluate partnership opportunities, and, ultimately, to guide the group's decision to join with an area hospital and form what would become a much larger integrated primary care network.

Looking into the future, the practice seemed to see two alternatives — remain independent, or merge in some manner with another entity. Although highly desirable, remaining independent would be extremely difficult. Even though the practice was well regarded in the community, it was losing patients as employers entered into managed care arrangements with which it was not affiliated. The community was the corporate home for a number of Fortune 500 companies as well as headquarters for several large insurance companies, and all of them were offering managed care insurance to their employees.

Early planning meetings after the arrival of the practice administrator convinced the remaining shareholders of the importance of responding to the needs of the community, and that managed care was quickly replacing fee-for-service medicine. If the practice did not want to be left behind, it needed to accept managed care contracts. The decision to accept managed care required a major change in philosophy, but because the practice was among the first primary care groups in the community to accept managed care, it doubled the number of patients seen by its physicians in one year.

With managed care comes the additional responsibility of managing the care. Successful though the practice was with its managed care contracts, it found the costs of office overhead increasing, in part because of the increased costs of paperwork. Costs had also increased due to governmental regulations from the Clinical Laboratory Improvement Act and the Occupational Safety and Health Administration. However, the group had secured a line of credit in order to purchase a new computer system, which enabled it to manage resources more efficiently. The number of patients increased, and the group began to think of ways to continue expanding.

Problems of physician recruitment and retention emerged. An employee physician left to join a larger primary care group that could offer him a much higher salary with a much better benefit package and, additionally, very little call responsibility (only 1 weekend in 16 as compared to 1 in 4). With increased recruitment competition from multispecialty clinics, hospitals establishing primary care clinics, and insurers recruiting in the area, it became evident that a smaller practice would have difficulty remaining competitive in the market for qualified family physicians. Lifestyle demands of the candidates included:

- High salaries, signing bonuses, and performance bonuses
- Reduction in call responsibilities
- Increased benefit packages, insurances, disability, profit sharing, and pension plans

It appeared that a small group simply could not command the capital resources necessary to fund desired growth. The increased stress and overwork on the part of the remaining physicians caused by all these forces led the practice to consider alternatives to independence.

Decision Alternatives

A number of merger and acquisition opportunities were surfacing in the area and in surrounding communities, which had formerly been havens for fee-for-service medicine and fiercely independent physicians. A large multispecialty group had embarked on increasing its extremely short-staffed primary care department by setting up multicommunity primary care satellite clinics and "groups without walls." One local hospital had created an elementary management services organization. Another local hospital had made inquiries into primary care practice acquisitions to enlarge its base of urgent care facilities, much to the disdain of its medical staff. One other distant hospital had begun making inquiries about expanding its network further into the suburbs, where the population base was expanding. Several insurers had begun setting up clinics in direct competition with established practices, in order to serve not only their own patients but others as well. All of these entities, with their ability to access capital for expansion, were successful in recruiting new family physicians, and they all wanted to talk with the primary care practice as it was the only well-known group in the area with a track record in managed care. The practice felt that potential partners would look favorably at its experience and conclude that its success made it a less risky partner when committing their capital for the acquisition and expansion of the group.

The Process

It was necessary for the group to make inquiries not only externally, but internally as well. How could it decide if one of these potential partner entities was an option? How could it manage the emotions these internal inquiries would evoke? The responsibility for focusing the physicians' attention on the process of decision making, rather than leaping quickly to a decision, fell to the administrator. Physicians, facing increased economic pressures, might enter questionable arrangements; but ultimately, the final decision needed to be acceptable not only to the group but to the community as well. The physicians needed to be made aware of the pitfalls that could result from a decision based on emotion and the promise of big dollars for the sale of the practice. The process of carefully implementing a merger or affiliation often is overlooked by the individuals or groups involved. Importantly, medical groups often have little, if any, experience in successfully implementing new ventures such as this.

The process began with "vision meetings," in which everyone was asked to respond to questions that would serve as a guide for initial discussions.

1. Where would you like to see yourself personally and professionally in one year? In five years?

2. Where would you like to see the group in one year? In five years?

3. What strengths would our group offer to a new group or partner?

4. What are the weaknesses of our group?

5. What goals would you like realized out of an affiliation? Please rank these in order of importance to you.

6. What do you see as possible barriers to an affiliation?

7. What are you willing to give up if we pursue an affiliation?

8. What are you not willing to give up under any circumstances?

9. If you had to make a decision today, what type of partner opportunity would you think best for the group and why?

All of the physicians were asked to think of their personal goals as well as those of the group in order to identify areas of potential conflict. Analysis of the group's strengths and weaknesses proved a useful forerunner to discussions of the group's short- and long-term goals related to an affiliation. It was especially valuable to rank these goals in order of importance to the physicians, to note potential conflicting goals, and to address all concerns before they became issues or barriers to later discussions. Potential obligations that would be necessary to participating with a new entity were discussed in detail as the physicians considered what they were, or were not, willing to give up in a new relationship. Here again, consensus was extremely important as the practice looked to the various kinds of affiliation under consideration. All offered differing levels of rewards, depending on the required levels of commitment and obligations, and the group could ill afford to make mistakes. It became imperative that the physicians have a clear understanding of the obligations each entity might require of them.

The issue of control (i.e., what they would give up versus what they would not) centered around what one physician termed a grieving process. Getting through this process was necessary for both individuals and the group, if the group was to get on with other important issues. To many, the grieving process was perceived as accepting the loss of control of an individual's practice. The physicians identified three factors as contributing to this sense of loss.

The first was the depersonalization of medical care. Patients were shifted from one medical group to another when employers changed coverage from one managed care company to another. The continuity of care, so important to the physicians in their medical school years, seemed to be breaking down. Patients seemed not to care if they had a permanent primary care physician, as long as they received care in a timely manner, and the care rendered was appropriate. Furthermore, patients were coming to the practice because their insurers said they must see primary care physicians. Patients could no longer visit their specialists when they wanted, and they often voiced their resentment at not being allowed to do so.

The second factor contributing to the physicians' sense of loss was that treatment decisions in managed care were based on what insurers would allow. Decisions were often made on the telephone by someone other than a physician. What, where, and when procedures would be allowed, as well as the lack of choice of providers led to the third factor adding to the sense of loss: erosion of the referral base with whom the physicians felt comfortable.

The feeling of loss of control was very real to the physicians, but the group needed to accept it in order to accept the concepts of managed care. Many physicians felt that, if this is what the future held for physicians, it made sense to give up the physical control of the practice. Why not give up the worries and hassles of practice management and concentrate on the delivery of health care? This frank discussion brought out much emotion, but it facilitated a basic acceptance of feelings and permitted a shift in focus toward setting new personal and practice goals.

The physicians went on to discuss the type of affiliation they might prefer and to identify any prejudices or preconceived notions they might have with respect to one or more opportunities. Certain areas of difficulty appeared. For example, prior experience with the style and attitude of managers in one of the area hospitals was discussed in order to determine whether or not it might hamper, in the physicians' opinions, a true sense of partnership with their group practice.

One of the key elements in the visioning process was the review of pertinent literature regarding mergers and affiliations. Key articles were distributed, and these served as the bases for considerable discussion. The literature documented the experiences of other groups as they moved through the decision-making process. Factors leading to failure were identified, such as copying the competition, merging with a distrusting partner, expecting miracles, and not knowing when to quit.

This strategic vision process was time-consuming but was the most important phase of the project. It helped the group reach consensus about pursuing next steps. The administrator's role was both to facilitate the sharing of ideas and, more important, to assess physician commitment to the decisions that were made. At the end of this process it was clear the group could no longer maintain independence.

The next stage in the process was to develop a set of criteria, based on the previously identified personal and professional goals, with which to measure potential partner opportunities. The group decided that any affiliation worth consideration should offer:

1. An improvement in lifestyle: proper vacation time, allowance for continuing medical education, a less stressful environment, an increase in benefit levels, and allowance for outside activities such as school or community teaching.

2. Protection for key staff members, including the practice administrator, an increase in benefits for these staff, and protection of current employee physician contracts.

3. Access to capital resources for the recruitment and retention of qualified physicians; the purchase of new equipment and renovation of offices; and possible expansion to a new satellite facility.

4. Interest and investment in community and patient care programs, for instance, a geriatric program, which the area desperately needed. The group did not want dollars taken out of the practice and the community left without assurance that some would be reinvested.

5. No disruption in referral patterns. Fears of specialist retaliation or exclusion were very high in the physician community due to moves to vertical integration and exclusion of specialists in this process.

6. Physician control of the day-to-day practice of medicine, with shared responsibility for quality assurance programs. The medical staff wanted shared governance in issues directly affecting the office, with provision for expansion of roles if desired.

7. Timely decision processes.

8. Maintenance of the group's identity. Name recognition was important, as the practice name was well respected in the community.

9. A fair purchase price based on acceptable standards with no hidden loopholes.

10. An exit plan, should the merger or acquisition not work out, fair to both sides, depending on level of investment.

Strategic questions, based on these criteria, were developed for use in discussions with each potential partner:

1. What is the mission of your organization?

2. What are your short- and long-term goals in this opportunity, and how do you see the practice adding to the achievement of those goals?

3. How will the group's physicians, administrator, and current staff be included in this venture? Will there be guarantees for current employee physician contracts?

4. Describe the decision-making processes for accessing capital for growth and new programs.

5. How is governance structured or how will it be structured? What role will the group's physicians and administrator have in decisions affecting the group, such as selection of additional physicians?

6. How much control will the physicians have in the day-to-day practice of medicine? In furthering the development of quality assurance programs?

7. Will the identity of the practice be preserved?

8. Identify the key people in your organization and their experience in ventures of this kind.

9. How do you see this merger or acquisition benefiting the community?

10. What will be the responsibilities and obligations of the physicians in the new venture, and how will the physicians be evaluated?

11. How will you help the practice communicate this merger to members of the physician community, given that community's current political climate of hostility to vertical integration?

Responses to these questions would assist in understanding the motives of a potential partner and in seeking common goals between the two entities. Potential deal breakers, points on which the group could not compromise, would be identified early on. For each meeting, an agenda and specific questions were prepared. The group's team included key people who came to the meetings on time, with clear information and decision-making authority. The team felt that being well prepared would confirm the group's commitment to the idea of affiliation.

Implementation

Responses to the strategic questions were graded much as on a report card, allowing a rank to be assigned to each prospective partner. Participants were allowed to comment and express opinions regarding the accuracy of the response. The team evaluated the participants from other organizations, and considered their demeanor representative of level of commitment and competence of those organizations. In one case, the team's only contact was a marketing representative who could neither speak for his organization nor provide answers to the team's questions in an acceptable manner — suggesting that this potential partner was not looking for a partner. A composite rank of seven to ten points on all responses identified organizations with whom the team wished to continue discussions. Middle-rank responses, four to six points, did not eliminate a potential candidate but meant that those responses would need substantial additional investigation.

To obtain further information, particularly any negative feedback regarding possible partners, the administrator and the attorney interviewed references — key administrators and physicians in other practices. This was a critical step in the investigation process. Physician responses were considered extremely important. Questions included:

1. Are you pleased with the new venture? Did it meet most of your expectations? Which expectations were not met, and why?
2. Did the venture fit with your strategic plan?
3. Does the venture deliver what it promises? In a timely manner?
4. If you had it to do over, would you? Why, or why not?
5. Do you know any group that is unhappy or has left the venture?

Potential partners proved to be quite willing to provide references. Supporters of potential partners were more easily found than critics, but the team found both. Most physicians who had entered into new arrangements were extremely candid and freely discussed both positive and negative aspects of their particular venture. It was not surprising to hear that many groups had not done any homework and had signed agreements that put them in vulnerable positions with virtually no role in day-to-day operations. The team viewed these negative comments as cautionary and examined them in detail. A simplified force-field analysis chart (see Table 1) assisted with internal discussion, illustrating all of the forces for and against a successful affiliation.

Table 1. Force-Field Analysis Chart

Current Situation	Desired State
Physician animosity or fear of any hospital-physician integration	Acceptance of affiliation

Driving Forces	*Restraining Forces*
Spiraling costs of overhead	Lack of physician understanding of integration issues facing primary care physicians
Lower physician incomes	
Decreasing enjoyment of lifestyles due to call schedules, more management responsibility	Fear of loss of control
	Fear of peer pressure
Penetration of corporate style of practice	Inflexible mindset against
	Fear of specialist retaliation against
Loss of business to insurers, etc.	
	Lack of participation in managed care, fear of cut in fees
Increased demands of managed care	
Need to access capital for recruitment and retention of physicians, satellite expansion, and new programs	Fear of personnel cuts, loss of favorites
	Fear of hospital retaliation
Shared risk	Fear of loss of identity
Access to quality assurance management	

A significant recurring theme in this analysis was fear of peer pressure. The community did not perceive vertical integration positively, and this was a major concern to potential partners as well as to the practice. There was also serious discussion as to whether the two local hospitals would express animosity, as they might be threatened if they were not selected as partners. The effect of the group's decision on other primary care groups that faced many of the same problems was also seen as potentially threatening to these hospitals.

As the investigative process uncovered negatives, the team discussed them with key administrators from potential partner groups. One potential candidate investigated the practice, including sending out "patient shoppers," who called, made appointments, and were seen by the group's physicians. That organization also prepared a report card on the practice, reinforcing the impression that this potential candidate was indeed interested in the practice as a group, and not just as another purchase. Both organizations were interested in a good fit.

Decision

The team narrowed the field of potential partners to two candidates. One was a local hospital seeking to acquire the practice to form the beginning of a primary care network. The other was a more distant hospital seeking a joint venture to expand its primary care network.

The team began serious negotiations with the local hospital by requesting a letter of intent that indicated a mutual commitment to pursue a venture. All issues, including agreement on purchase price and governance, were to be settled within 30 days. Both parties pledged absolute secrecy during this period. However, during this 30 days, a number of other administrators were made aware of the project, and the board of directors of the hospital proposed a vote. Physicians on the hospital board then communicated their extreme unhappiness with the idea to other physicians in the community, and all confidentiality was lost. Negative letters arrived in the practice's office via fax, and physicians from the group were stopped in the halls of the hospital and accused of selling out. It was determined that key administrators did not have board support as they had suggested, nor was confidentiality as was pledged. Further, it was learned that the hospital was also entertaining other affiliations, thus calling into question the administration's good faith.

Several weeks later, the group began serious negotiations with the other hospital. Within 15 days of the practice's receipt of a letter of intent, formal papers establishing the joint venture were drawn up, and the negotiation was successfully concluded.

Questions for Discussion

1. What were key elements of the process that led to a successful negotiation and conclusion of an affiliation?

2. What negative consequences might have occurred if the group had not developed and used a process for decision-making?

3. Describe the role of physicians and administrators in this process and how they did or did not contribute to its success.

Managed Care

Public Managed Care in Easternville
A Case of Opportunities

by Carolyn Watts Madden

A number of states have made extensive use of experimental or demonstration programs as a means of moving cautiously down the path of health care reform. Experimental programs appeal to policymakers for a variety of reasons. First, as the interior designers of public policy, experimental programs make policy visions concrete. Second, they can allow innovation to occur in small, protected steps.

The most important function of such experiments may be to facilitate innovation and guide its next steps. Since a primary deterrent to innovation is fear of the unknown, reducing this fear reduces the deterrent. Experimental programs can generate useful information that reduces uncertainty (e.g., knowing the utilization behavior of a particular target population reduces the uncertainty about the costs of covering this population). They can create a protective environment in which innovative industry practices (e.g., capitation contracts with physicians unused to capitation) can evolve at a comfortable pace. In this environment, administrative systems to manage these innovations (e.g., management information systems) can be developed and tested. Finally, experimental programs can create provider linkages that extend beyond the program, both in time and in scope (e.g., contracts between plans and physicians to cover experimental populations can be extended to cover commercial populations at the end of the experiment).

The Setting

Easternville is a town of about 300,000 located in an otherwise rural area of Washington state. One of the two dominant sources of medical coverage in

Easternville is a medical bureau that has been serving the community for over 35 years. The medical bureau, Eastern Physician Services (EPS), provides traditional indemnity insurance coverage for roughly 30 percent of the local population, paying the claims of most of the area's 400 physicians.

EPS primarily serves small and medium-sized businesses, but it also has contracts with two of the region's large employers and offers two types of individual policies. To date, all of its physician contracts have been fee-for-service contracts, through which EPS pays a predetermined percentage of physicians' established fees.

The other major player in the insurance market in Easternville is an old, respected closed-panel, managed care organization with a market share almost equal to that of EPS. With the exception of the salaried primary care providers on the staff of the closed-panel plan, most physicians in Easternville are in solo practice. In recent years, however, the number of small groups has increased, and EPS has secured contracts with the two large multispecialty clinics in town.

The Opportunity

Washington's legislature recently created a state program that offers subsidized insurance to families and individuals with incomes below 200 percent of poverty. The program was authorized as a five-year demonstration program administered by an independent state agency. The benefit package is fairly basic. Prescription drugs, vision care, and mental health services are excluded, and there is a 12-month preexisting conditions exclusion for all services except maternity. The state is restricted to contracting with managed care organizations for no more than 20,000 enrollees in at least five counties across the state. The agency administering the new program, the Basic Health Plan (BHP), has issued a request for bids. Successful bidders will receive a capitated monthly payment for each individual enrolled, in an amount negotiated between the plan and the state. Plans must provide the specified benefit package and accept all individuals who qualify for enrollment. That is, a plan may set an upper limit on how many people it will enroll, but it must enroll on a first-come, first-served basis.

The Response

Senior staff at EPS voiced some interest in bidding on the BHP. They knew, however, it would be a significant challenge, particularly since the organization had never operated under a negotiated capitated contract before. In the end, EPS decided to bid, for two primary reasons. First, a few key players, both in the administration of EPS and among Easternville's physician community, felt a social responsibility to participate in the new program. Because EPS dealt largely with employed populations, it had little opportunity to serve low-income residents of Easternville. While some of EPS's member physicians did serve low-income and uninsured patients in their practices, the BHP was seen as an opportunity for EPS to expand this activity and to receive reimbursement for the services provided. Second, most people involved in the decision realized that movement to managed care practices, while slower in Easternville than in other parts of the state, was inevitable. Therefore, participation in the experimental BHP afforded an opportunity to develop some experience in this unfamiliar method of operations early and in a relatively low-risk environment.

In preparing its bid, EPS invited 300 member physicians to participate in the BHP product. These providers were selected based on EPS's years of experience with area providers, and a cursory analysis of fee schedules and practice patterns as reflected in submitted claims. Nearly all of the 300 providers, both primary and specialty care, accepted the invitation and entered into contracts with EPS. Providers were offered a fee-for-service contract with a small percentage of total payments to be set aside and refunded at the end of each year based on the group's performance. Three of the area's four hospitals were also offered fee-for-service contracts. No formal utilization management was prescribed, either for inpatient or outpatient services. EPS placed a limit of 2,000 on the number of enrollees it would accept in the first year.

Easternville's closed-panel plan also submitted a bid, and both were awarded BHP contracts at different rates as negotiated by the two organizations and the BHP. Eligible enrollees in Easternville were allowed to choose either plan, with the premium differences between the two absorbed by the BHP; enrollees paid the same premium for either plan.

Good local publicity and strong demand for the program resulted in rapid enrollment in the BHP. EPS met its limit of 2,000 in the first nine months of operations. The first year's experience was good. The adverse selection that many plans feared did not materialize. In fact, BHP enrollees appeared to have slightly better experience than most groups plans, and EPS showed a modest profit in this product line at year's end.

Extension

After the second successful year of BHP operations, EPS was presented with another opportunity. This time, the state's Medicaid program was soliciting organizations willing to enter into capitated contracts to serve the individuals receiving Aid to Families with Dependent Children (AFDC). This program, termed Healthy Options (HO), operated under a waiver of federal Medicaid rules and offered substantially different terms than the BHP. First, the AFDC population eligible for HO was different (very low income, and primarily mothers and babies), and larger (total AFDC eligibles in the Easternville service area was about 20,000). Second, the HO program was mandatory for those eligible, whereas the BHP had always been a voluntary program. Third, the BHP was a small agency that had demonstrated its sensitivity to the needs of contractors.

Further, because of slower than expected enrollment in other areas of the state, budget problems had not yet hit the fledgling program. On the other hand, Medicaid was housed in a huge agency full of rules and regulations, including constraints imposed because of the federal funding partnership, with a reputation for much less sensitivity to the needs of providers, and little experience in dealing with managed care plans.

Again EPS decided to participate, as did the closed-panel plan. EPS offered a separate contract to essentially the same panel of physicians that had BHP contracts. This time, however, primary care providers were offered capitation contracts for their services, with a separate budget for fee-for-service payment of specialty and hospital claims. The change in contract was motivated primarily by heightened concern about utilization. However, it was in large measure the two years in the BHP program that gave both EPS and its providers sufficient experience and courage to proceed in this fashion.

The first year of HO was rough. AFDC recipients who were enrolled in EPS were unfamiliar with its systems and procedures. In particular, they were unused to primary care physicians serving as gatekeepers. Rather, they were accustomed to seeking primary care from the emergency rooms of hospitals at any time of the day or night, without appointment, and to choosing when and from which specialist they would seek care. A number of the women were accustomed to using an obstetrician/gynecologist for routine primary care services.

Physicians and hospitals were also overwhelmed by the changes brought about by HO. Referral procedures were not well understood. In a fee-for-service environment, such misunderstandings were awkward, but had little financial effect. In a capitated environment, the financial consequences were large. The effect on some emergency rooms was another complication. A number of Easternville's emergency rooms derived a substantial portion of their income from primary care treatment of Medicaid patients. The loss of this revenue to the two participating managed care plans generated anger and dislocation.

EPS persevered, and during the second year of operations, undertook a number of administrative changes to address problems encountered during the first year. Extensive education campaigns were launched, aimed at both enrollees and providers. As many offices as possible automated referral systems so that patients did not have to carry with them a referral slip — which during the first year had often been misplaced or forgotten. Another education campaign was aimed at the staff of local emergency rooms. In addition, EPS offered a triage fee to the emergency rooms for funneling nonemergent care back to the primary care physician. Membership cards were reissued with the name and phone number of the enrollee's primary care physician, so that when the patient arrived at the emergency room with a nonemergent problem, the primary care physician could be contacted.

By the end of the second year, emergency room visits by HO enrollees in EPS had been reduced by 25 percent, with office visits up by an offsetting amount. Patient satisfaction, measured by responses in focus group sessions, had improved, although there was still some discomfort with limitations on specialty referrals and the stigma associated with being a welfare recipient — which, a number of people asserted, affected the quality of care they received. Provider satisfaction was also high, with a number of primary care physicians reporting that their revenue from HO exceeded 100 percent of fees from prior years. Access, as measured by the number of physician practices open to Medicaid patients, had improved greatly. Of roughly 150 primary care providers in EPS's Healthy Options list, only 17 had closed their practices to new patients. This was a substantial improvement from pre-HO days, when few if any providers accepted new Medicaid patients.

From Public to Private: Further Extension

As EPS prepared for its fourth BHP year and its third HO year, it created a new division to oversee its three managed care products — including a new commercial managed care product (EPS Care), which it planned to market in competition with the closed-panel plan. The commercial product expanded on the experience with both the BHP and HO. Again, primary care provider contracts were capitated, and many of the operating systems, including a new management information system, created for use in the public programs were expanded to accommodate the needs of EPS Care. Since EPS had begun to expand beyond Easternville's urban area by creating new provider linkages for its BHP and HO products, the commercial venture was able to start with this broader market area.

Questions for Discussion

1. How did the experience with experimental programs affect the nature and pace of innovation at EPS?

2. What was the consequence of the size of the BHP program for EPS's decisions? What might have happened if HO had come along first?

3. What was the role of administrative interest and leadership in the decision to participate, and what were the ultimate consequences of participation?

4. How might a seriously negative experience with the BHP have affected future EPS decisions?

5. How might the commercial product affect future offerings of the BHP, which was ultimately converted to a permanent, statewide program, and HO?

Sound Med
A Case Study in Community Relations

by Janet Piehl

In September 1994, two members of the citizens' advisory committee of the board of directors of Sound Med lodged a formal complaint, charging Sound Med with disproportionately serving the more affluent communities of the Seattle metropolitan area and not serving the traditionally underserved neighborhoods. A special task force composed of employees from the organization, as well as community representatives, was convened to study the problem and develop an action plan.

Background

In the late 1960s, a group of health care providers in Bellevue, Washington, decided to try, as a social experiment, providing health care coverage to patients who paid for their services up front with a small monthly fee. The group called itself BellCare, and agreed to be paid an annual salary, with any profit being funneled into a program to provide services to the poor not covered by the relatively new Medicaid program.

After the Health Maintenance Organization (HMO) Act of 1974, BellCare changed its name to Sound Med, retained its not-for-profit status, and began a program of slow expansion into the rural and suburban areas of King, Pierce, and Snohomish Counties. Sound Med chose to focus upon less populated areas, feeling that such areas needed greater access to health care than the cities.

In 1982, however, a young pediatrician, Jennifer Hawkins, began to push the HMO to open centers in Seattle, arguing that much of the urban area was underserved. She eventually won over the board of directors, and in 1985, Sound Med opened its first center in downtown Seattle. Two years later, it opened a second center on Capitol Hill, followed in 1988 with one in Ballard. Sound Med opened its most recent Seattle center in 1990, in the University District.

As of September 1994, Sound Med, still headquartered in Bellevue, had enrolled over 250,000 members throughout King, Pierce, and Snohomish counties. Sixty percent of its centers operate as staff-model HMOs, with the physicians receiving an annual salary, and the remaining 40 percent operate on a group-model, with the physicians receiving a contracted capitation fee for each member enrolled in the panel. Members prepay for all services; the company makes a profit when its members are healthier than average, supplying an incentive to provide cost-effective preventive care. Each member signs up with a primary care physician gatekeeper who manages all of that patient's health needs and coordinates specialty referrals.

Demographics

Sound Med has enrolled 17 percent of the total Seattle population, with over 20 percent penetration in four neighborhood districts: Central, Southeast, Lake Union, and Green Lake (see Exhibit 1). It has enrolled fewer senior citizens than reside in the community at large; 12 percent of its members are over age 65 versus 15 percent for the entire city of Seattle. However, it has enrolled a higher proportion of children less than 16 years old, and women ages 16 through 64 — 18 percent and 55 percent of enrollment, versus 15 percent and 51 percent for the city, respectively. Both groups are traditionally higher utilizers of health care services than men in the 16 to 64 age cohort (see Exhibit 2).

Exhibit 1. Sound Med, Seattle Market: 1994 Penetration Rate by Neighborhood District

District Neighborhood	9/94 Enrollment	Population 1990	Rate Penetration
Central	7,324	28,611	25.6%
Southeast	10,836	46,707	23.2%
Lake Union	6,004	26,803	22.4%
Green Lake	1,121	5,315	21.1%
Duwamish	7,262	36,675	19.8%
Southwest	12,559	70,555	17.8%
Downtown	3,433	19,507	17.6%
Northeast	11,331	68,675	16.5%
Ballard	8,536	52,694	16.2%
Northwest	7,043	51,407	13.7%
Capitol Hill	4,483	35,302	12.7%
Queen Anne	5,720	45,393	12.6%
North	2,812	28,695	9.8%
Total	88,464	516,339	17.1%

Source: City of Seattle Office for Long-Range Planning, *Census 90: Population Changes in Seattle, 1980–1990*, April 1991.

Exhibit 2. Sound Med, Seattle Market: Age and Gender Distribution by Neighborhood District

Neighborhood District	< 16 years	16–64 years	65+ years	Male	Female
Southeast	24%	62%	13%	48%	52%
Duwamish	22%	65%	13%	50%	50%
Central	19%	67%	14%	49%	51%
West Seattle	18%	65%	16%	48%	52%
North	14%	70%	16%	47%	53%
Ballard	14%	67%	19%	47%	53%
Northwest	14%	69%	17%	47%	53%
Northeast	12%	75%	13%	50%	50%
Queen Anne	11%	72%	17%	47%	53%
Lake Union	9%	81%	10%	49%	51%
Capitol Hill	9%	77%	14%	52%	48%
Downtown	3%	74%	23%	60%	40%
Total	15%	70%	15%	49%	51%

Source: City of Seattle Planning Department, *Census 90: Sub-Area Profiles, 1990*, February 1993.

Note: Between 1991 and 1993, the City of Seattle redefined its neighborhood districts in reporting 1990 Census data. Therefore, the neighborhood districts in Exhibits 1 and 2 are not strictly comparable.

Task Force Assignment

The board of directors of Sound Med asked the Director of Planning to convene a task force to address the concerns of the citizens' advisory committee and develop an action plan to present to the board. The task force consists of the members shown in Table 1, with the Director of Planning chairing the meeting. (See Appendix for descriptions of each of the members.)

Table 1. Task Force Members

HMO Administrators	Health Care Providers	Community Leaders
Director, Planning	Physician	Deputy Director, Neighborhoods
Director, Marketing	Nurse Practitioner or Physician Assistant	Community Activist

Membership and roles are to be assigned prior to the convening of the task force, and members are to come to the meeting prepared to discuss the questions that follow. Special consideration is to be given to issues of access to medical care, demographics, public relations, business decision making, governance, finance, and Medicaid reimbursement and structure.

Questions for Discussion

1. What are the primary issues to the members of the citizens' advisory committee who launched the complaint? To you as a member of the task force?

2. What will you include in your action plan? How will you assign tasks to committee members as laid out in your action plan?

3. How will you implement your recommendations? How will you pay for them?

4. How will you ensure that all voices are heard, within the task force, the organization, and the greater community?

5. How can Sound Med better position itself to avoid similar complaints in the future?

Appendix to Case 22. Task Force Members

Director, Planning — Task Force Chair

The Director of Planning is responsible for all strategic and long-term interests of the HMO, including but not limited to expansion planning, business planning, national, state, and local governmental regulations and policy, competition, and new business ventures. In addition to basing expansion plans on need and demographic analysis, the director tries to site Sound Med centers in "neutral" areas. These centers are located in areas that are accessible to public transportation, but not necessarily situated directly in underserved neighborhoods. Thus, they provide access to those members who rely on public transportation, without alienating members who would not travel to the heart of undeserved neighborhoods.

Director, Marketing

The Director of Marketing represents the company's customer service and public relations interests, as well as sales and marketing.

Physician

This role may be ascribed to either a primary care or specialist physician. The primary care physician has a strong interest in public health issues and believes strongly that primary care physicians are well trained to handle most medical problems. The specialist, on the other hand, believes that primary care physicians are qualified to manage less complex cases, but is concerned that primary care doctors do not always refer complex cases soon enough. In addition, the specialist feels threatened, both professionally and personally, by health reform proposals that may restrict specialty care.

Nurse Practitioner or Physician Assistant

This mid-level practitioner feels that mid-levels provide excellent, cost-effective primary care services, particularly through fostering communication with patients and counseling them in behavior modification. This caregiver feels that physicians sometimes forget that they are treating people, not diseases, and that mid-levels are better able to provide the flexibility that a changing American health care system needs.

Deputy Director of Neighborhoods, Mayor's Office

The mayor's office is interested in boosting its "urban village" concept in rebuilding and revitalizing the urban core. The Deputy Director of Neighborhoods is pushing for Sound Med to be a major participant in this plan.

Community Activist, Receiving Medicaid Benefits

A recipient of governmental assistance, the community activist is tired of being treated as a second-class citizen. Sound Med is proud of having its highest penetration rates in the Rainier Valley and South Central Seattle, some of the poorest sections of the city. However, the community activist knows that this penetration rate is based upon people actually counted in the census and does not include many of the residents of the poorest neighborhoods.

CASE 23

Managed Care Meets the Ivory Tower

Providing Ambulatory Mental Health Services at an Academic Medical Center

by John C. Blanchard

Northern Medical Center combines Northern Hospital and Northern Medical School, which merged in 1939. The medical center's clinical faculty and hospital-based ambulatory services provide 500,000 ambulatory care visits per year. Its 800-bed teaching hospital provides 222,000 inpatient days of care, and its combined workforce is 9,000, or approximately 20,000 total covered lives.

Like many major employers, Northern Medical Center has experienced rapid increases in health benefits costs in recent years. Cost-escalation factors have included the referral of employees and dependents off-campus to high-cost providers, and a general lack of controls over benefits utilization. For example, ambulatory mental health benefits claims paid grew by almost 70 percent from 1990 to 1991 alone — even as inpatient benefit expenses continued to rise. Total health benefits claims expenses were expected to continue an upward trend if no incentives were implemented for cost-effective use of health benefits dollars.

Nationally, ambulatory and acute mental health care services are increasingly being designed, purchased, delivered, and evaluated in terms of a managed care model. Alternative ambulatory service settings, utilization management tools, risk sharing, and fee discounts are usually considered integral parts of a managed mental health care system. Within these systems, there are practical and ethical needs to provide options to employees as to where they receive health care services, and to ensure patient confidentiality.

Under traditional health benefits plans, however, relatively unchecked access to expensive mental health care services has contributed significantly to increased costs. Northern Medical Center's strategic and financial interests will be served to the extent that it can provide its own workforce with managed mental health care, and encourage its workforce to use, when appropriate, a specific panel of mental health care providers.

Northern Medical Center's total employee and dependent health benefits costs have been a major, growing operating expense. Total employee and dependent health benefits claims paid, combining Northern Hospital and Northern Medical School figures, exceeded $18 million in 1992 and were projected to grow 25 percent per year.

Paid benefits claims for mental health services alone ranked as the second-leading health benefits expense for Northern Medical Center in 1992, accounting for over 10 percent of total institutional health benefits dollars, and were growing at an estimated rate of 20 percent per year. This rate of increase in behavioral health care benefit expenses caused increasing alarm.

New Program

The medical school's department of psychiatry was requested to propose a managed mental health care program in which the department would be a preferred provider for ambulatory mental health services for the Northern Medical Center workforce. The department, in turn, proposed that Northern Medical Center and the department together create health benefits incentives for employee and dependent use of a select panel of providers for inpatient mental health care services.

In addition, the department was charged with the design of specific utilization management services for Northern Medical Center, to be phased in over a period of two to three years. This approach was envisioned to allow many affected parties to gain experience with the new program gradually, and therefore enhance the likelihood of program success. From the outset, the department also planned to solicit preferred provider contracts with major employers throughout the region.

The general parameters of the managed care program include two separate contracts: one between the department and Northern Hospital, and one between the department and Northern Medical School. The vision for the managed mental health program is to achieve positive, measurable institutional effect (e.g., cost savings) without requiring radical changes in health benefits design, restrictions on consumer choice, or significant administrative burden.

Departmental Capacity

The department provides physician-level and master's-level diagnostic and therapeutic psychiatric and behavioral health services on an ambulatory basis in its offices within Northern Medical School and in three acute care units situated in Northern Hospital. The department has also increasingly provided corporate liaison services with the health benefits staffs of a growing number of area employers who refer patients to Northern Medical Center; area employers have indicated increasing interest in developing managed care contracts with the department for meeting the behavioral health needs of their workforce.

Total outpatient visits to the department increased from 6,187 to 8,150, or 31.7 percent, between fiscal year 1989 and FY 1992. While 51.3 percent of mental health outpatient visits in FY 1990 were residents of the immediate county, 55.6 percent were local residents in FY 1992, suggesting an increase in ambulatory market share. During this period, psychiatric admissions at Northern Hospital increased by 2.6 percent, but due to a decrease in length of stay, total inpatient days of care decreased by 6.6 percent.

Within the psychiatric faculty, two physicians also held master's degrees in health services administration and kept abreast of trends in managed care contracting. Thus, with a well-developed professional staff, growing outpatient activity, and a geographically wide patient origin mix, the department felt well positioned to provide expanded clinical and management services.

Traditional System

Although the coverages within the Northern Hospital employee and dependent benefits plan were generous in comparison with other area employers, incentives had been introduced to encourage use of medical center resources, including psychiatric services. For example, outpatient psychiatric care provided at the medical center was covered 100 percent as compared to 80 percent if provided elsewhere, following the annual deductible. Pastoral counseling was also covered 100 percent after the deductible. There was neither control over actual charges demanded by other providers (e.g., outpatient therapy fees), however, nor were utilization management tools part of the mental health benefits program.

Northern Medical School employees and dependents enjoyed relatively less generous health benefits. For example, outpatient psychiatric care was covered 50 percent regardless of the provider, after the annual deductible was met.

Referral Process

Historically, Northern Medical Center employees and dependents were free to choose from a wide range of professional and institutional mental health facilities and services. Employees and dependents who sought psychiatric or substance abuse treatment often referred themselves to services elsewhere, even out of state, with few limitations and little oversight.

Employees and dependents also sought mental health care services through the employee assistance program (EAP). Employers typically sponsored EAPs to encourage cost-effective, early treatment interventions and to ensure user confidentiality. Operating on an evaluation-and-referral model, Northern Medical Center's EAP provided referral assessments for individuals, couples, and families seeking psychiatric, psychological, and substance abuse treatment.

Although the EAP claimed to provide a limited number of mental health referrals, it maintained unusually wide latitude in recommending treatments and providers, with little accountability for cost-effectiveness or quality outcomes.

Mental Health Claims Expense

According to data from Northern Hospital and Northern Medical School, combined paid claims expenses for mental health rose from $1.64 million in 1990 to $1.97 million in 1991 or 20.1 percent. Components of these expenses included a 6.6 percent increase in combined inpatient claims expense, and a 68.6 percent increase in combined outpatient claims expense — clearly a figure that was cause for alarm.

Several factors contributed to increases in utilization of ambulatory mental health services, including virtually unlimited access to those services, competitive marketing efforts, and financial disincentives for effective cost controls. Northern Medical Center management and medical staff expressed widespread concern that little control over quality care was present in choices of mental health care service providers.

Referrals of employees and dependents to other ambulatory and acute care providers represented a significant opportunity cost to Northern Medical Center. Extreme variations in ambulatory charges, number of encounters, and acute care lengths of stay at other facilities contributed to runaway employee and dependent mental health claims expenses and sapped resources from other possible uses.

With respect to acute care, in 1991 only 16.8 percent of hospital employees and dependents admitted for psychiatric care were admitted to Northern Hospital. In the same year, only 15.8 percent of medical school employees and dependents admitted for psychiatric care were admitted to Northern Hospital.

Program under Implementation

The medical center implemented a managed care contract between the department and both Northern Hospital and Northern Medical School to become a preferred provider for mental health services for all employees and their families. Goals specified for the program are to improve the availability, utilization, and evaluation of cost-effective, high-quality employee and dependent mental health services.

The department will continue to provide all professional diagnostic, therapeutic, and consultative services available in its existing programs. The department will not alter the scope of services presently available to Northern Medical Center employees and dependents. A medical center-wide internal marketing effort to communicate changes in health benefits design was initiated in 1993 regarding the managed mental health care program.

Patient Confidentiality

Confidentiality is often paramount in the choice of referral for mental health care services in particular, and the department remains highly sensitive to patients' rights to privacy and confidentiality. With respect to ambulatory services, the department proposed in 1993 that additional off-site locations be explored to provide employees and dependents with additional means of maintaining privacy while seeking mental health services such as individual, couples, or family therapy.

For example, the department proposed providing certain outpatient services at an off-campus complex with flexible hours and scheduling. Policies prohibiting consecutive appointment times for employees and dependents were planned, in order to decrease the likelihood of unrelated Northern Medical Center employees and dependents meeting inadvertently at off-site locations. This was viewed as an important practical and symbolic effort to serve the interests of patients' privacy.

The department also proposed that a panel of regional acute care providers be created to preserve nonmedical center options available to employees and dependents for acute mental health care services. This panel has been developed, such that employees and dependents from either institution would be treated at a mutually discounted rate.

Utilization Management

The department was designated to provide utilization management for all mental health services as a mechanism to ensure the appropriateness of referrals. Review functions will be performed by a departmental committee of midlevel and physician faculty. It is critical that the utilization management function be performed with objectivity to avoid conflicts of interest. Medical staff liability insurance was to be obtained for utilization management services, as required by current state insurance department regulations.

It was anticipated that the cost of utilization management staff support, and physician-level faculty for utilization management services, would be subsidized by Northern Medical Center as a combination of per-case payments and a percentage of cost savings in relation to historical mental health claims expense. Contractual specifications also require use of clinical practice guidelines, not only to ensure objectivity but in support of outcomes research.

Quality assurance data reflecting utilization of mental health services by employees and dependents under the preferred provider relationship, including self-referrals, EAP referrals, and referrals through other channels, will be carefully monitored and disseminated to appropriate Northern Medical Center parties to help assess the effectiveness of these changes.

Since a reduction in payment for clinical services is a central feature of the managed mental health program, and the provision of utilization management services represents a significant resource investment, the department is assuming an unprecedented degree of risk for both efforts.

Conclusion

Northern Medical Center has taken several innovative steps to improve its management information systems, implement changes in employee health benefits, explore new methods for contracting with major purchasers, and improve its managed care posture generally. Northern Medical Center has the opportunity in 1996 to benefit from both lower employee and dependent health benefits costs and predictable revenues through a managed mental health care program.

Fee schedule discounts, benefits design changes, and new utilization management efforts are key components of the medical center's effort to reduce institutional health benefits costs while increasing the efficiency of clinical services. These initiatives will promote the use of internal resources (i.e., health benefits dollars) to purchase other internal resources (i.e., health care services for employees). The department believes this can be accomplished without affecting the availability of alternative options or sacrificing patients' rights to privacy and confidentiality.

These efforts may be widely perceived as a valuable investment in the medical center's single most important resource, its workforce. This managed mental health care model has potentially valuable applications for academic medical centers across the United States in the 1990s.

Questions for Discussion

1. What marketing and communications steps should be taken to ensure that the medical center's workforce views the new program positively?

2. Will community-based providers of mental health services be affected by the new preferred provider plan? If so, should this concern the medical center?

3. Can a major employer provide limits on mental health services without jeopardizing employees' freedom of choice, or need for confidentiality?

4. Is the local corporate community likely to respond favorably to a new managed care program for mental health services — one that was piloted at an academic medical center?

CASE 24

Mid-State Group Practice Ventures into Managed Care Contracting

by Keith Boles

Health care reform movements, together with the activities of the marketplace to reform the delivery of health care, regardless of the actions of the various governments, have had a major effect on the consideration of risk. In earlier times, when hospitals received cost-based reimbursement and indemnity insurance paid hospital and physician charges without asking for accountability or efficiency, risk was not discussed or important. Any risk associated with the illnesses and injuries of individuals, and the associated utilization of health care services, was borne by the payers — government and insurance companies. Costs were distributed throughout the population in the form of taxes or increased premiums. While this process may have achieved the objective of equity in access to health services, it certainly did not encourage efficiency, or even effectiveness, as the various parties involved all reacted rationally to the incentives provided to them. The issue of risk, and who bears that risk, is central to the emerging health services environment.

In this earlier reimbursement environment, patients initiated the health services encounter with the physician due to the presence of some medical condition. The physician then performed those services that the physician felt were appropriate, or in some cases were desired by the patients and billed the patients' insurance company. The insurance company paid the physician whatever was billed and the insurance company collected sufficient insurance premiums from the patients to cover all physician and hospital bills. The providers bore none of the risk associated with how often they saw their patients, whether or not these patients were hospitalized, how many services were utilized in the provision of health care, or the costs associated with any of the services provided.

In the capitation environment, much of the risk associated with patient utilization of health services is shifted onto the providers. It is imperative that the providers have sufficient information and creativity to adjust to this new environment.

It is this environment in which the Mid-State Group Practice (MSGP) finds itself. The MSGP has been approached by The Health Plan (THP) regarding participation in a managed care program for THP enrollees. MSGP consists of ten primary care physicians. This is the first such contract that they have considered, and the physicians are wondering how they should approach the negotiations. They know that their operations must somehow change, but they aren't sure how. THP has said it will pay $33.72 per month for each enrollee choosing a physician in MSGP. An additional 15 percent of this amount is to be placed in a risk pool. This risk pool will be distributed to the physicians in the event that a surplus exists at the end of each contract year. A surplus will exist as long as referrals and hospitalizations are not above the actuarial norms for the enrolled population. If a shortfall occurs in this risk pool, MSGP will have to reimburse THP for up to 15 percent of the deficit.

MSGP is located in an urban area with a population of close to 2 million. Managed care has been relatively slow to penetrate into the marketplace there. However, the management and physicians of MSGP have seen the writing on the wall and are anxious about their first managed care contract. They are concerned about the amount and types of information that they need to be able to respond appropriately to the offer from THP. The physicians realize that the managed care organizations are trying to control costs by increasing physicians' awareness of the financial implications of their treatment decisions. One way of increasing this awareness is to place physicians at financial risk for their treatment decisions.

THP has been in existence for five years, has grown to have a total of 100,000 enrollees, and is seeking to expand its provider base. It has a reputation in the local market for being an aggressive negotiator and for making a reasonable profit for its stockholders, while still providing quality health care services.

MSGP must examine the revenue risks and operating risks of THP's offer. Revenue risks are assumed to be risks that have an effect only on revenues, while operating risks have to do with operations — utilization rates and associated costs. With the fee-for-service patients that MSGP has historically seen, the profitability position of the group improved both as more patients were seen and as more procedures were provided per patient encounter. The physicians in the group have seen their take-home distributions increasing at the rate of 8 percent to 10 percent per year during each of the past five years. They are concerned that this trend will not continue, especially after hearing anecdotal evidence from their colleagues who have more managed care contracts.

The physicians of the group are very concerned with what will happen, in terms of their practice styles, their cost of operations, and their income levels, under the proposed contract. They want to identify the various risks with which they must deal, the types of information that they must have to make a rational decision regarding the appropriateness of the proposal, the variety of options available to them to survive and prosper in the managed care environment, how to handle a situation in which fee-for-service patients are being seen at the same time as capitated patients, what they can do to manage or otherwise handle the risks that THP will attempt to place on them, and how many of these risks they are willing to accept. Table 1 presents workload measures per physician for both MSGP and THP. Table 2 is MSGP's revenue-and-expense statement.

Table 1. Workload Measures per Physician

MSGP

CPT-4 Code	Description	RVUs/ Month	Frequency/ Month
99212	Office/Outpatient Visit, Est., Level 1	67.58	100.11
99213	Office/Outpatient Visit, Est., Level 2	139.64	140.09
99214	Office/Outpatient Visit, Est., Level 3	34.06	22.87
99215	Office/Outpatient Visit, Est., Level 4	22.92	9.74
59410	Obstetrical Care	23.01	9.10

THP

CPT-4 Code	Description	RVUs/ Month
99212	Office/Outpatient Visit, Est., Level 1	73.25
99213	Office/Outpatient Visit, Est., Level 2	151.42
99214	Office/Outpatient Visit, Est., Level 3	57.60
99215	Office/Outpatient Visit, Est., Level 4	32.21
59410	Obstetrical Care	12.17

**Table 2. MSGP Statement of Revenues and Expenses,
Prior to Distributions**

Revenues	$3,521,980
Nonphysician Expenses	
Administrative supplies / services	69,310
Building / occupancy	243,560
Furniture / equipment	60,120
Information services	75,190
Insurance premiums	109,030
Laboratory	135,670
Medical and surgical supplies	168,170
Nonprovider benefits	217,860
Nonprovider salaries	867,860
Promotion / marketing expenses	15,810
Radiology / imaging	54,590
Total Nonphysician Expenses	$ 2,017,170
Total Nonphysician FTEs	43

Questions for Discussion

1. Develop the list of information that needs to be collected and analyzed before the group is able to give an educated response to the offer. Students will have to make some assumptions regarding the historical utilization rate of the MSGP patient base.

2. What are the key risks that MSGP will be accepting if it accepts a capitation contract?

3. What techniques could be used in the contracting phase to reduce the risk exposure to the physician group practice?

4. Is the capitation rate sufficient for this contract?

5. Should the group accept the contract?

Planning and Strategy

CASE 25

Care Transitions Across Settings
A Challenge for One Hospital Administrator

by Charles E. Hawley and Stephanie A. Simon

John Rogers sat back in his chair with a smile on his face. He had just returned from a meeting of the board of directors of Middleton Community Hospital. At the meeting he had announced that the hospital had won a sizable managed care contract for 10,000 enrolled lives, including a significant number of Medicare enrollees. The contract had been awarded in major part due to the hospital's successful efforts in becoming an integrated delivery system through the development of a physician-hospital organization (PHO). John is pleased with the tremendous strides the hospital has made in developing the PHO. As he reflects on the events of the last year that have led up to this contract award, he feels vindicated. It had been hard work to convince many of his board members about the importance of integrated delivery systems, and now his efforts had paid off. Appointed to his first CEO position just a year ago, John has worked hard to get to this point in his hospital administration career.

Middleton Community Hospital is located in a two-hospital town in the West. The hospital has taken the lead in the community to become a successful player under health care reform. A major strategy has been to contract with primary care physicians through the formation of a physician-hospital organization capable of competing for managed care contracts. A leading primary care physician in Middleton had been hired to organize and direct the PHO. In order to retain and support the core business of providing inpatient acute care, creating and supporting linkages with the provider community was critical in the development of this network.

Under the PHO model, the primary care physician serves in the role of case manager and gatekeeper to specialty services. The case management component is particularly appealing to prospective managed care payers as a way of effectively managing costs. Realizing the importance of tracking cost data, the hospital had made considerable investments in the last year to upgrade the capabilities of the information system. As a result, the PHO administration has the ability to track and monitor high utilization and high cost cases in the hospital. This first large managed care contract signifies that the hospital has successfully entered the world of capitation. John feels Middleton Community Hospital has done the essential groundwork and is ready for managed care.

This focus on monitoring costs and improving hospital operations has also led to a substantial decrease in average length of stay. The development of clinical pathways — increasingly emphasized as a way to improve the efficiency of patients' care during their hospital stay — along with the ability to track and monitor costs have made the hospital more competitive in the market when bidding for new contracts. In addition, continuous quality improvement initiatives, such as the recent completion and analysis of a patient satisfaction survey, are under way.

John recalls how pleased the board had been with the financial reports during the meeting. Over the last year, with the impending cost pressures associated with market reform, the hospital had decided to divest itself of certain unprofitable operations, particularly in the area of long-term care. The hospital had owned a nearby nursing home and a hospital-based home health agency. These investments had been made when the hospital was pursuing a diversification strategy, but they had failed to achieve adequate financial returns. Consequently, the hospital leadership team, along with the board, decided to get out of the long-term care business. Instead, they decided to focus all of their efforts on building and nurturing the PHO relationship in order to protect the hospital's market share, and to ensure its role as a key player in the frenzied marketplace.

The Phone Call

As John reflects on the tremendous strides the hospital has made toward integration, he is interrupted by a phone call from his wife, Sally, who is noticeably upset. She has just received a call from John's sister, Karen, informing them that John's mother has had a stroke and is in the hospital in Wheaton, 300 miles away. John is shocked and concerned, relieved only by the fact that his mother is at Wheaton Medical Center, a facility with an excellent reputation. Despite his concerns about her health, John feels comforted in knowing she is in good hands. In fact, for the last year, he has modeled Middleton's efforts toward integration and clinical quality improvement after the work done by Wheaton Medical Center, clearly a leader in the region. John tells Sally that he's on his way home to pack a bag and will catch a flight to Wheaton that evening.

On his way to the airport, John can't help thinking about the last conversation he had with his mother. She had recently stopped taking her blood pressure medication because it was making her feel sick. This was of great concern to John, and he had pleaded with his mother to go see her family physician. She had refused, saying it would take too long to get an appointment that she considered unnecessary. John wished he had called the doctor himself, as his mother had had high blood pressure for many years and had experienced difficulty in performing some normal activities of daily living.

His Experience at Wheaton Medical Center

John arrives at Wheaton Medical Center to find his mother in the intensive care unit. He is somewhat surprised that his mother's long-time primary care physician has not been called. After he is assured that his mother's condition is stabilized, John finds himself bombarded with a number of questions from the clinical staff. He becomes increasingly frustrated as he attempts to answer their well-meaning inquiries concerning his mother's medical history and the availability of such documents as a living will. Initially, John is concerned that the clinical pathway calls for his mother to be discharged on the fourth day following her stroke. However, he is relieved to learn that she will qualify for admission to the hospital's rehabilitation unit. After talking to the nurse case manager on the rehabilitation unit, where he answers many of the same questions all over again, John feels assured that his mother is on the road to recovery. Telling his mother that he will be back as soon as he can, John returns to Middleton. Over the next few days, he hears about her rapid progress in rehabilitation and turns his attention to the mounting work he had left behind.

A few days later, as John is working at his desk on a contracting strategy, he places his daily call to his mother. He is surprised to learn that she has developed a urinary tract infection from her catheter. As a result, she has been transferred out of the rehabilitation unit, back to the medical unit. John had not known that his mother had been catheterized at the hospital, since she had never had a problem with incontinence. John can tell that his mother's emotional state has deteriorated, as she seems depressed and withdrawn on the phone.

His Experience with Home Care

Overwhelmed by matters at home and work, John is unable to return to visit his mother until she is scheduled to be discharged to home care. He and his sister, Karen, meet with the unit nurse to learn how to care for their mother at home. The nurse explains a complicated series of procedures that need to be carried out, involving the use of intravenous solutions and durable medical equipment. Both John and Karen leave the hospital overwhelmed at the extent of care they must provide for their mother at her home. John agrees to stay with his mother for the first week, during which several home care visits are scheduled.

John finds himself looking forward to the first home care visit, as he is struggling to meet his mother's needs. However, the first visit is distressing, as the home care nurse indicates that she is there primarily to assess his mother's needs and develop her care plan. While talking with the nurse, John becomes upset because he has to answer many of the same questions that he previously answered in the hospital. The nurse tries to calm John by explaining that the home care agency is not linked to the hospital's information system. Consequently, the agency was unable to access information from his mother's inpatient visit. Additionally, John is surprised by the minimal amount of information that the hospital discharge planner provided to the nurse assigned to care for his mother.

After taking care of their mother for a few days, John and Karen find the care required to be more intensive than they had imagined. Even with home care services every other day, John finds himself ill prepared to cope with the physical and emotional requirements in addressing his mother's needs. John is exhausted and drained. His mother appears withdrawn and unwilling to cooperate. He faces tremendous difficulty in even getting her out of bed. His mother complains that she is not feeling well and that her legs ache. After a couple of frustrating days, John is called away to urgent matters at work, leaving Karen to care for their mother.

Two days later, John receives a call from Karen informing him that their mother needed to be readmitted to the hospital for an elevated fever, dehydration, and possible blood clots in her lower legs. While their mother's condition has now stabilized, Karen is still upset: when she arrived at the emergency room, she was bombarded with all the same questions that John had faced. Does their mother have advance directives? Is she allergic to any medication? "Why do they have to keep asking all the same questions?" Karen asks. John explains that they have to ask these questions, but in the back of his mind he thinks there must be a better way. John, too, is frustrated by the lack of coordination of his mother's care, as she had left the hospital only two weeks earlier.

Nursing Home Placement

A few days later, John returns to see his mother and learns from the doctor that, because of the lack of improvement in her condition, she must be admitted to a nursing home. John is shocked and dismayed; he had never considered placing his recently active mother in a nursing home. Again, John thinks, if only something had been done to make sure his mother had taken her blood pressure medicine, maybe none of this would have happened. The discharge planner provides John with a list of nursing homes. John does not feel well equipped to make this decision for his mother. As he begins looking around, he is surprised by the out-of-pocket costs associated with nursing home care. It is all very expensive, and Medicare will cover the cost of her care for only a few days.

After his mother's discharge from the hospital, John helps her move into the nursing home he has chosen. Again she is reassessed, and again a care plan is prepared. John is frustrated as the nursing home staff begins to ask questions concerning his mother's medical history and advance directives. He is shocked when the admitting nurse shows him the discharge summary from the hospital: it simply reads, "Transferred to Nursing Home." No information from her prior hospitalizations accompanies her to the nursing home. Additionally, John is disappointed to learn that his mother will have a new primary care physician, as her family doctor does not make nursing home visits. At this point, his mother's health has deteriorated substantially. She appears lifeless and keeps saying over and over that she wants to go home. John assures her that he will return as soon as he can for a visit.

The Plane Ride Home — A Time for Reflection

On the plane ride home, John reflects on his mother's current state. He remembers her health and vitality just a few months ago, and wishes something could have been done to prevent what has happened.

To divert his attention and concern, John decides to catches up on his long-neglected reading file. He notices an article about a hospital's continuous quality improvement process on strokes, which details the success of this project in reducing the length of stay, thereby achieving considerable savings. Furthermore, the hospital is now realizing profits on this diagnosis-related group. In the past, John would have been excited about this approach. Now, however, some new and troubling questions begin to emerge. Does simply reducing the length of stay measure quality? Where are these patients going upon discharge? Are they being sent home to informal caregivers left to struggle without sufficient support? Who is monitoring care after discharge to ensure patients are getting better? Thinking once again about his mother, John wonders if any of the strokes referenced in the article could have been prevented. Would earlier intervention and follow-up of high-risk individuals have made a difference?

As John sits back in his seat, he begins to understand how limited his view of health care has been. He realizes how ill prepared Wheaton Medical Center and his own hospital are in caring for people with chronic conditions. In being so focused in the last year on enabling the hospital to contract in the new managed care environment, John lost sight of the need to manage individual care. He has the contract, but he lacks effective systems for managing the health of these newly enrolled populations.

John returns to his reading file and comes across an article about "managing care across the continuum." He begins reading with interest about the organizing principles in achieving a true integrated continuum of care — administrative restructuring, management and clinical information systems, capitated financing, and care coordination and case management to achieve continuity of care. John is impressed by how these ideas address many of the limitations in his own thinking.

As John begins to apply these concepts to his mother's experience, he sees how this continuum-of-care approach would address many of the problems he encountered. John is particularly excited with case management, which seeks to identify individuals at risk before more serious problems emerge. This concept would have been a great benefit to his mother, perhaps even preventing her stroke by carefully monitoring her medications.

John is also impressed with the idea of integrating information systems across sites. Since his mother's chart had been institutionally based, it was not surprising that she had been reassessed at every new site. Better coordination of information was clearly needed.

John's mother's care had not been properly coordinated: her long-standing primary care physician did not follow her course of care in the hospital or during home care. Additionally, there was no financial incentive for her doctor to see John's mother in the nursing home. Rather than receiving well-coordinated care with a systematic approach, John's mother experienced a series of isolated events. This need for care coordination was also painfully evident from John's own experience as primary caregiver after his mother's discharge from the hospital.

John thinks about all the bills from various providers and about how high the cost of treatment has been. Capitated financing could address much of this confusion, some of which arose from itemized lists of services, each stating, "This is not a bill."

As he thinks about ways Middleton Community Hospital might address these issues, John begins to feel excited. He recalls that a new administrative fellow is coming on board when he returns, and decides to ask the fellow to develop a briefing paper to assess the limitations of Middleton Community Hospital's current strategy, and to consider how the hospital can better work with other organizations in the community to develop a continuum of care. He wants the paper to address the fundamental issue of managing the care of an individual across care sites, looking for models around the country that have focused on care coordination and case management strategies. John hopes to approach the hospital leadership team with a strategy for becoming part of a continuum of care. This continuum will focus not only on contracting with providers but also on creating a system for managing the care an individual receives in different places and at different times during the course of an illness.

Questions for Discussion

1. What strategies can Middleton Community Hospital pursue to:
    - Identify and monitor high-risk individuals?
    - Coordinate care delivery across settings so that the individual does not experience a series of isolated events?
    - Enable the primary care physician to participate in care planning and treatment as an individual moves from one care setting to the next?

- Structure information systems so that patient information can be shared across settings?

- Provide more support for such informal caregivers as family and friends?

- Measure outcomes across settings, rather than simply being institutionally based?

- Create clinical and administrative structures that support coordination of care?

2. Which steps can the administrator take in the short term, and which strategies must be explored in the longer term?

Expansion of Hospital-Based Service Systems to Support a Satellite Clinic Network

by Linda Kay Horton

Hospital administration asked Kathleen Daly, until recently administrator of one of the hospital's 11 clinics, to guide the expansion of hospital-based support services. Hospital administration had decided that it would be more cost-effective to provide support services for its eight off-site clinics and three on-campus clinics through in-house departments rather than through outside vendors. Ms. Daly was charged with coordinating the hospital support departments' efforts to provide these services to the clinics.

In order to understand the challenge at hand, it was important for Ms. Daly to review the development of the clinic network and its relationship to the hospital support departments. Then, it was necessary to determine how the hospital's support departments could actually provide the level of service appropriate for off-site primary care clinics, since the hospital departments, while comfortable with the provision of services to centrally based, inpatient nursing units, were unfamiliar with the needs of the clinics. Careful discussion was necessary in order to overcome department heads' hesitation to alter their service standards.

History of the Clinic Network

In the early 1980s, the hospital determined that, in keeping with its mission to provide health care to the poor and underserved in society, it would pursue a grant to build and operate a primary care clinic in an economically depressed, inner-city neighborhood. This became the hospital's second clinic, the first being the family practice residency clinic located on-campus at the hospital.

Throughout the decade, the hospital added clinics to the network, at an average of one every 18 months. Some of the clinics were practices that the hospital acquired. Others the hospital developed, which required constructing facilities and recruiting physicians.

Of the 11 clinics in the network, three were based in office buildings on the hospital's central campus. Two of these on-campus clinics included specialists. The third was the family practice residency clinic. Nine clinics were exclusively primary care and located within a 20-minute drive of the hospital. Board-certified family practice physicians predominated in the network. Many of them had graduated from the hospital's residency program.

In all but one case, the hospital owned and operated the clinics, and the physicians were hospital employees. In the final case, an affiliated clinic had an operating agreement with the hospital, but the physicians remained independent practitioners. All physicians within the network used the hospital primarily for inpatient work and for outpatient diagnostic work not available in the clinic setting.

Prior Linkage between Clinics and Hospital Support Departments

In late 1989 and early 1990, the administrators of the hospital emphasized developing mechanisms for hospital support departments to provide services to the clinic network. Two chief operating officer positions were created at the hospital level to support this process. Ms. Daly filled one of these positions, after having spent four years as manager of two of the off-site clinics.

Prior to 1989–1990, certain support departments had provided services to several of the clinics. However, few service programs were offered consistently throughout the network. In addition, service standards were generally focused toward the traditional, inpatient customer of the support departments. It was up to individual clinic managers to determine how they might piggyback on the existing service standards to address the needs of their clinics. Clinic managers rarely worked together in this process. Thus, a hospital department's provision of services to a particular clinic tended to reflect the clinic manager's ability to influence the head of the support department.

Consequently, the services being provided to the clinics were a patchwork. In some clinics, the hospital department provided the service. In other clinics, the manager used an outside vendor. Even when several clinics used a hospital department for the same general service, the type of service and the degree to which it was provided varied. The use of outside vendors involved similar variation, since the manager of each clinic selected its vendors and established its service standards and contract prices.

Service and Quality Effectiveness

This amalgam of support services led to a host of administrative and operational difficulties. Primary among these was expense management. Each clinic manager developed the least costly structure for support services that he or she could. However, this effort toward cost reduction was constrained by how much time the manager wanted to devote to the process and by how much he or she knew about the alternatives. This methodology had been acceptable prior to hospital administration's decision that these services would be provided by hospital support departments. That decision eliminated this clinic-by-clinic approach and gave rise to the project assigned to Ms. Daly.

Prior to this project, each clinic manager had had the burden of monitoring the appropriateness and quality of the various services provided to his or her clinic. This was a time-consuming process. Furthermore the effectiveness of this process with respect to any specific service was limited by the individual manager's understanding of that service. Clinic managers were thrust into technical areas for which they had little background or training. For example, they needed to understand the appropriate preventive maintenance schedules for the clinic's heating/ventilation/air conditioning system and the correct cleaning substances to be used to eliminate the biohazards in a dirty procedure room. Learning curves were often steep.

An additional area of difficulty was presented by the hospital's need to satisfy the requirements, regulations, and standards of several regulatory and accrediting bodies. Since the clinics were departments of a hospital accredited by the Joint Commission on Accreditation of Healthcare Organizations, they were also subject to JCAHO standards. The variation in service standards and the number of vendors used did not facilitate compliance with such standards and regulation. When compliance was attained, the explanation of procedures was often difficult, and documentation was poor.

In addition, if the needs of a clinic changed after selection of a support vendor, the manager had to negotiate directly with the vendor to adapt services to the new needs. This meant that, on many occasions, the clinic manager was serving as a contracting officer without the benefit of legal support.

Managers' difficulty in managing the variety of support services in their clinics contributed to a very stressful climate. Additionally, the lack of consistency among clinics with regard to service vendors and service standards hindered collaboration within the clinic managers' group on issues of service management.

All of these problems negatively affected operational effectiveness, as clinic managers struggled to manage support services and to operate all other areas of their clinics. Managers indicated that they often spent one-third of their time each week obtaining, implementing, monitoring, and evaluating the provision of support services to their clinics. This resulted in time away from management of other clinic functions, such as patient service, physician productivity, patient flow, accounts receivable, employee supervision, and physician relations. It became clear that the use of hospital support departments, if correctly designed, implemented, and managed, would allow the clinic managers to do a better job filling the roles for which they were hired.

Scope of Revisions to the Service Delivery System

Once the hospital's administrators completed their cost-benefit analysis and decided that the clinics should use the hospital support departments, it was important to itemize and set priorities for the services that the hospital departments could provide and, if the departments were already providing services, how they could be improved. Ms. Daly led this effort.

For several services, the support departments had no experience in working with the clinics. Consequently, the departments needed to do significant developmental work to offer them to the clinics. In other areas, departments were already providing some support to at least one of the clinics. For these services, it was necessary to refine standards and to expand operations to include all clinics. Finally, there were a few services that the hospital was not equipped to provide. A more effective process for contracting with outside vendors needed to be developed for these services, in order to capitalize on the purchasing power of the hospital and clinic network.

Improve Services Provided by Hospital Departments

The hospital had traditionally provided some support to the clinics in four areas: materials management, communications, risk management, and maintenance. Ms. Daly reviewed the services these hospital departments provided to the clinics and identified the opportunities for improving them.

Materials Management

The materials management department included all contracting, purchasing, processing, and distribution functions for supplies, equipment, services, and forms. The department's support to clinics consisted of delivery of linen, supplies, and interoffice mail; purchasing; contracting; vendor selection; and product standardization. The materials management department head was a long-term employee of the institution and had been involved with the clinics from the early stages in their history. While his department provided a fairly complete array of services to the clinics, a problem existed in that materials management provided these services according to hospital, rather than clinic, specifications.

Also, while most of these services worked fairly well for the clinics, key problems existed within each service area. Solutions had to be developed before the entire clinic network could rely completely on the hospital for these supports. For example, a clinic would not receive its requested linen if the hospital's linen use had exceeded expectations — regardless of whether or not the clinic had placed its order in advance of the hospital's order. The hospital would appropriate the clinic's linen. Another example of inadequate service was the fact that, although supplies were delivered to the clinics by truck, a routine schedule had never been developed. Thus, inventory control was difficult in the clinics. Another example is that interoffice mail for the clinics was delivered on the supply truck and was frequently lost among the boxes of supplies. Also, the truck did not arrive at the clinics on a daily basis, rendering interoffice mail unreliable, as a frequent, predictable, and consistent scheduling for delivery of linen, supplies, and interoffice mail delivery was necessary.

With regard to purchasing, contracting, and vendor selection, the hospital's purchasing department was willing to support the clinics and, in fact, had designated a clinic buyer at an early point in the network's growth. The remaining challenges were: (1) to assure that the clinic buyer understood clinic requirements; and (2) to develop communications between clinic managers and the purchasing department to facilitate vendor selection, contracting, and purchasing.

Product standardization proved to be the most difficult issue to resolve relative to materials-management, even though the hospital's purchasing department was supportive and eager to be of assistance. The difficulty came, in part, from a lack of understanding on the part of the hospital concerning clinics' supply needs. A greater obstacle came from clinic managers and clinic physicians, who were used to being able to order their own preferred supplies rather than buying a standardized item in bulk.

In all of these instances, clarifying service needs and forming work groups proved to be useful in problem resolution.

Communications

Hospital administration had always expected the clinics to use the hospital's print shop for forms and other printing, the communications department for marketing, and the purchasing department for photocopier leasing. The communications department hired a person for clinic marketing and provided considerable support. There was, however, a difficult period of learning as the department improved its understanding of techniques that would be effective for promoting the clinics.

Photocopier leasing was well supported by the hospital. Printing, however, proved to be a difficult service for the hospital to provide to the clinics. The shop was so disorganized and inefficient that the clinics — as well as other hospital departments — risked being without necessary forms for long durations due to print shop mismanagement. For many essential forms, the clinics used outside vendors even though the print shop had expressed a clear willingness to support the clinics. Frank discussion and definition of service expectations led to improvement of these issues, although not to their complete resolution.

Risk Management

Risk management was one support service that the hospital had provided to the clinics consistently and in a generally satisfactory manner. Included within this area were such services as infection control, quality assurance, employee health and assistance programs, malpractice and liability insurance, and legal advice. Difficulties did exist in making quality assurance programs and studies applicable to the clinics. In addition, infection control programs had to be revamped to pertain to the special needs of the clinics. Nonetheless, the hospital reliably provided expertise and assistance to the clinics for risk management endeavors.

Maintenance and Repairs

Although the hospital had complete facilities engineering and maintenance departments for the physical plant, none of their services was available to the clinics. The only support for maintenance and repairs in the clinics was through the purchasing department's negotiation of service agreements for major equipment, such as x-ray units and laboratory analyzers. There was no problem with this purchasing department support, but the clinics felt that much more needed to be done for them through the facilities department.

The facilities department head was fairly new to the institution and had inherited a department in disarray due to limited resources and the ineffectiveness of the prior manager. Included among this department head's responsibilities were the maintenance of a hospital facility with a main building dating from the early 1900s and the management of numerous construction and renovation projects on the main campus. Consequently, the idea of adding nine off-site clinics to his list of concerns was difficult for this department head. The development of service standards, however, made it possible for him to provide maintenance and repair support to the clinics without detracting from his on-site responsibilities.

Develop Services by Hospital Departments

There were a number of services that the hospital provided to itself but neglected to extend to the clinics. Prior to working with the heads of the support departments to develop systems for providing these services to the clinics, Ms. Daly needed to identify the deficiencies. The services that were not provided to the clinics generally fell under department heads who already provided other services to the clinics or had some interest in doing so. Thus, the process established for refining existing services also worked well for developing of new services, since the same individuals were involved.

Materials Management

The purchasing department historically neglected inventory control for the clinics. It made no attempt to establish par stock levels or to simplify the ordering process. At the conclusion of this project, the ordering process had been extensively revised and simplified. The warehouse began to stock frequently ordered clinic supplies. Inventory control still rested with the clinics, but discussions were under way with materials management to determine how this might be automated.

Communications

No hospital department provided direct support to the clinic managers for the selection, installation, operation, or maintenance of phone systems. In addition, the clinics had no fax machines, and as stated above, interoffice mail delivery was unreliable. Finally, all clinics had to make their own provisions for mail services and postage meters. At the end of this project, all but two clinics had fax machines. All clinics had favorable postage meter lease rates or were able to use the hospital's mail room. Also, several clinics had used the hospital's telecommunications expertise to facilitate the selection and installation of new phone systems.

Risk Management

Despite the fact that the clinics received certain risk management services from the hospital, they remained without assistance in at least two areas of risk management and quality assurance: safety and security, and instrument sterilization. The clinic managers were expected to arrive at solutions for any problems in these two areas. Again, considerable improvement had taken place by the end of the project. Quality assurance, infection control, and safety programs had been modified to meet the particular needs of the clinics. Instrument sterilization was planned for implementation within the next several months.

Maintenance and Repairs

The hospital departments did not provide the clinics with support for repair and installation of equipment, preventive maintenance, or building maintenance. Each clinic manager made arrangements for these services to the extent that he or she was able. This project brought about equipment and facility preventive maintenance programs. In addition, a maintenance employee was scheduled to visit each clinic once a week to perform minor repairs and installations.

Continue with Outside Vendor for Service

The hospital was not in a position to provide a final set of services to the clinics. These included janitorial, information processing, and mail services. Although the hospital maintained a housekeeping department, a data processing department, and a mail room, these departments could not feasibly assume responsibility for the clinics because of logistics and the special needs of the clinics.

For information processing, the clinics needed to remain independent from hospital-based patient accounts systems to maintain control over accounts receivable and billing operations. Also, data processing had not been an item included in the mandate from hospital administration, although it was clearly expected that the clinics would work with the hospital's data processing department to explore interfaces among systems.

Equipment, transportation, staff, and funds were not available to enable the housekeeping department to assume cleaning responsibilities at the clinics. However, two years after this project, the hospital provided janitorial services to the clinics.

For mail services, it was deemed inefficient to have U.S. mail arrive at the hospital's mail room for distribution to the clinics when the postal carrier could deliver mail directly to the clinics. Thus, the centralization of mail services was not pursued further.

Process for Revising the Service Delivery System

The process to modify or provide support services needed to be a collaborative one that emphasized communication between department heads and clinic managers. Mutual goals needed to be identified to ensure that changes could be implemented. Finally, the process had to support the effective delivery of services rather than political maneuvering. Using these premises, Ms. Daly developed an implementation plan that was applied separately with each of the involved service departments.

Implementation Plan

The first step of this implementation plan was the selection of work group participants, including representatives from the clinic managers' group and the service department head. A chairperson was designated from among these participants. Staff from the clinics and the service department were also often involved in work groups. Other hospital departments were involved in the process if they had either tangential or substantial involvement in the provision of a service. For example, the purchasing department could not be effective in improving turnaround times unless the delivery truck, which was operated by the warehouse, traveled to each clinic on a routine schedule.

Once a work group was established, the desired service was defined through the establishment of service standards. Service standards included such matters as when the service would be provided, how frequently, by whom, to what degree, with what equipment or supplies, and under what conditions. These standards also stipulated supervisory authority and reporting mechanisms. In several instances, service standards consisted of two or three statements. In one situation, a standard extended to three single-spaced pages.

Once service standards were developed, the head of the appropriate support department committed the department to meeting them. The clinic managers' group also agreed to the standards, since a support department could not be expected to provide effective service delivery if the demands were changed without a process for discussion, or if each clinic had a different expectation.

On occasion, the support department found it needed additional or different resources to provide the service to the clinics according to the identified standards. If this occurred, the support department head prepared and presented budget requests to the hospital's administrators. Representatives from the clinics joined in these presentations on request.

Once resources were arranged, the development of policies and operating procedures commenced. Again, collaboration was key in this process. Neither the clinic managers nor the support department head was able to dictate policies and procedures. Instead, these were drafted, discussed, revised, and redrafted. At all times, the work groups focused on what was realistic and possible. Timelines and start dates were intentionally conservative. Also, depending on the circumstances, introduction of the service was either staged, simultaneous in all clinics, or pilot-tested. The work groups continued to meet throughout the implementation process to resolve any problems that arose. Once the service was fully established, evaluations and revisions were ongoing.

This process was followed with all of the services except those that were to remain with an outside vendor. The difficulties encountered in the process varied with each service. Many of the problems were anticipated, but a number of major issues were not foreseen and delayed the provision of some services.

Problems Encountered

Among the problems encountered were politics, differing service expectations among clinics, confused lines of authority, resource limitations, and organizational ineffectiveness. Political problems most often appeared as a struggle for control over a particular service by two or more department heads. If allowed to continue unchecked, these problems would have clouded the development of service standards, policies, and procedures. However, because hospital administration's mandate was clear that support departments were to provide services to the clinics, most department heads moved out of this phase quickly.

The clinic managers were not immune to this type of wrangling, either. Several managers felt that services provided to their clinics should be under their control. Because this control was not the intended outcome of the process, the clinic managers had to develop relationships with service department heads in order to communicate their concerns to them.

Confused lines of authority did prevail with respect to certain services. This was, in all probability, the organizational deficit that allowed political maneuvering initially. For a number of services, it was not clear who had ultimate budgetary control and operational responsibility. For example, the clinic managers budgeted for certain services (e.g., facilities maintenance) but allocated or transferred these costs to the support department providing the service. The clinic manager had no involvement in the determination of the amount he or she was to transfer and no authority to hold the support department accountable for the service standards. It took a number of discussions among department heads and clinic managers to find a common basis of communication and to develop a consensus about the level of services to be provided for the predetermined transfer amount. Even then, tension remained, until a realignment in hospital administration placed the clinics and the support departments under the same administrative head. Then, communication and cooperative problem solving among support department heads and clinic managers improved.

The clinic managers had learned early in the project that they had differing expectations of desired services. Consequently, in addition to the planning and implementation processes outlined above, the clinic managers, as a group, had to spend significant amounts of time together to arrive at agreement about service standards. Because the clinic managers had formed an effective working group during the two years prior to this project, they were able to use established problem-solving skills to arrive at consensus.

In some cases, resource limitations precluded the development of the ideal support service program for the clinics. For example, it was determined that interoffice mail would be best handled via a daily courier service to all clinics rather than on the supply truck. Funds were not available for acquisition of a vehicle for an in-house courier program, and daily use of an outside courier service was found to be too expensive. Consequently, the focus was then shifted to solutions for the loss of interoffice mail when it was sent via the supply truck. Fortunately, within one year, a courier system was adopted for the clinic network, with twice-daily delivery and pickup.

Finally, organizational ineffectiveness prevented the effective establishment of some of the services to the extent planned in this project. For example, problems continued with the print shop's turnaround times. Thus, clinics continued to resort to outside vendors in order to obtain urgently needed forms. This occurred despite reasonably good efforts on the part of the involved department heads to identify service standards and to provide routine, consistent printing support to the clinics. In such matters, the clinic managers have learned how to provide objective feedback to the support department head and how to leave it to him or her to resolve the management issues.

Results

As a result of this project, support services to the clinic network by hospital support departments improved considerably. All services that had existed prior to the project were enhanced, and most absent services were established. Service standards and procedures were clearly articulated, and served to provide a strong foundation for a cooperative working relationship between the clinics and the hospital service departments. In addition, several services provided by outside vendors were identified as ones that could be brought in-house in the future, such as maintenance, janitorial, and courier services. In addition, the hospital laboratory began to complete laboratory tests for the clinics, a support service not envisioned earlier.

The satellite clinics are more efficiently operated as a result of this project. The clinic managers are able to devote their energies to managing their clinics rather than to coordinating support services. It is beyond the scope of this case to provide sufficient analysis to make a direct link between the financial performance of the clinics and the completion of this project. However, an example of the clinic managers' increased opportunity to focus on clinic operations may be seen in the significant reduction in days in accounts receivable for all clinics and in the improved cash-collection ratios for most of the clinics. Turnover rates among clinic staff have also declined in the two years since the events of this case. These facts may reflect improved management by clinic managers and the fact that a large portion of their time has been turned from the management of support services to the management of core clinic operations.

An added benefit of this project has been the enhanced visibility of the clinics within the hospital and the improved understanding and respect among hospital department heads and clinic managers.

Recommendations and Reflections

Any satellite clinic owned by or affiliated with a hospital could embark on its own effort to use the hospital service departments for its support needs. However, the support departments in large institutions are complex. In addition, they have a long-standing history of serving on-campus in-patient departments. Consequently, changing systems to support off-site ambulatory care facilities requires a long process.

Upon reflection, the length of time necessary to implement the provision of services to the clinics by the hospital's support departments was surprising. While many of the heads of support departments were enthusiastic and flexible, the lead time required to establish communication channels and to identify the clinics' needs and service expectations was substantial. Time was also required to overcome clinic managers' trepidation about giving up autonomy and control over certain functions.

Considerable momentum is necessary to overcome the inertia inherent in a complex and bureaucratic organization, such as a major medical center. Additionally, despite comprehensive cost-benefit analyses, a project such as this will encounter unanticipated expenses. Department heads have to be prepared to explain to the hospital's administrators why additional funds are necessary to implement their mandate.

In making recommendations to others undertaking a similar task, it is suggested that the project begin with clarification of: (1) priorities, (2) sources of funding, and (3) lines of authority and control. Otherwise, several months will be spent in the politics of the situation. Also, an administrative mandate is helpful and may, in fact, be necessary. However, if administration mandates an action, it also needs to have in place a method for evaluating department heads and managers in relation to that mandate. Delays were encountered in this project until department heads realized that administration was serious about the implementation of the changes they had articulated. Without such clarity, a project may come to a halt when middle managers encounter the organizational and operational difficulties of serving off-site facilities. It should also be acknowledged that a project such as this will uncover weaknesses and areas of ineffectiveness on the part of managers and department heads. Administrators must be willing to deal with those issues.

Creativity, flexibility, and humor are recommended for surviving an overhaul of service delivery systems. Effective communication skills are also imperative. If all of the talents of the management team are brought together in an effective process, the results will be well worth the investment.

Questions for Discussion

1. What organizational weaknesses led to the service problems between the hospital and its affiliated clinics?

2. In a fully integrated organization, what management principles might be applied to help avoid some of these problems?

3. How would you use continuous quality improvement practices to resolve these hospital-clinic service questions?

4. Can you identify some generic differences between hospital and clinic executives that might contribute to the problems described?

5. Conflict over priorities is a typical problem in complex organizations. What recommendations do you have for the CEO in order to help him or her minimize these conflicts?

CASE 27

Planning Facilities in a Managed Care Setting

by Katie Ricklefs, Patty Belson, Susan Flautt, and Patricia H. Mintz

In 1990, Dr. Gallstone, chief of staff of Santo Domingo Medical Center, and his medical staff faced a major challenge. Santo Domingo, a 120-bed community hospital with integrated medical offices, is part of a large multihospital health maintenance organization. Membership had grown modestly in the Santo Domingo area, but the organization had not kept up with its expanding facilities' needs. Consequently, space for medical offices and ancillary support services (e.g., laboratory, imaging, pharmacy) was severely strained on the campus. Appointment wait times were increasing, member satisfaction was dropping, physicians were doubled up in offices, and the patient care staff were increasingly frustrated. As an elected chief of staff, Dr. Gallstone felt he had only a short time in which to develop a plan to address the problems.

Part I

Santo Domingo is one of 15 hospitals in a two-million-member health maintenance organization. Because of rapid growth in the last three years, fueled by low rate increases and a robust economy, the organization had been challenged to finance an aggressive capital program. Planners estimated that over a ten year horizon, the HMO would need to invest $3.5 billion in facility expansion, renovation, and replacement projects to support the two million members. With increased pressure to provide care in lower-cost settings, which required supporting technologies, the major capital requirements were for additional outpatient services, especially in the primary care areas.

Dr. Gallstone knew that his expansion recommendations would exceed the $500,000 capital threshold requiring approval from the organization's central facilities planning committee. This group consisted of senior executives and representatives from the medical facilities responsible for authorizing all major capital investments. He had heard from other chiefs of staff that presenting recommendations to the facilities planning committee was known as "running the gauntlet." He knew that his request would come under great scrutiny.

The Santo Domingo Marketplace

Santo Domingo Medical Center is located in one of the wealthiest metropolitan communities in the ten counties included in the health maintenance organization's service area. As shown in Tables 1 and 2, the population in the area immediately surrounding the hospital is older, relatively affluent, and growing slowly. However 20 miles further north is a rapidly growing, much younger set of bedroom suburbs. The system planners projected that most of the future growth for Santo Domingo will come from these smaller communities to the north.

However, growing congestion in the north and south suburbs has gradually increased the travel time between the suburbs and the medical center. Convenience and easy access remain especially important to the affluent, well-educated population, as does excellent service.

Table 1. Projected Membership Growth

	1994	1995	1996	1997	1998
Santo Domingo, southern service area	120,000	121,000	121,500	122,000	122,500
Santo Domingo, northern service area	65,000	73,000	83,000	95,000	110,000
Total Santo Domingo membership	185,000	194,000	204,500	217,000	232,500

Table 2. Physician Office Requirements

	1994	1995	1996	1997	1998
Physician office requirements* for combined service area	123	130	137	146	160
Available physician offices at Santo Domingo	87	87	87	87	87

*Physician office requirements are based on a member to physician (and physician office) ratio of: 660 members per physician office. Midlevel providers (e.g., nurse practitioners) are allocated half the office complement of physicians.

While the main growth is occurring to the north, the medical staff have a strong desire to remain integrated on or near the existing Santo Domingo site. The primary care physicians feel that high quality care can best be provided with close proximity to specialist colleagues for timely consultations and easy access to nursing staff in order to address questions and problems. They believe this allows a more timely discharge for their patients, which is an important cost factor as well. Thus, the primary care physicians, as a group, express grave concerns about the loss of either continuity of care or proximity to their inpatients should a remote satellite be developed.

Options
With a team of planners, real estate staff, and selected medical and administrative staff from Santo Domingo, Dr. Gallstone identified four alternative approaches:

1. Build new office space on the existing campus
2. Lease adjacent office space in the community
3. Reconfigure existing space and expand hours of operations to gain additional required capacity
4. Develop new medical office space in the emerging population center

Contracting for primary care services in the community was not considered because it ran counter to a critical organizational tenet of the Santo Domingo medical staff.

Questions for Discussion
1. What information would you require to evaluate these options?
2. What criteria would you use to rate the options?
3. On what basis would you select one option over another?
4. What values would be of highest importance to the Santo Domingo medical staff as they provide input to the decision?
5. What values would be of highest importance to the members of the health maintenance organization?
6. What values would be of highest importance to the members of the facilities planning committee in their decision making?

Part II

The planners and Santo Domingo staff completed an evaluation of all four options, based on both quantitative and qualitative data. Their findings are shown in Table 3.

Concurrently, real estate and facilities construction staff determined that two of the options had to be eliminated for practical reasons. Option 2, leasing office space, was not feasible because, after an extensive real estate search, no available lease space was identified in the community. Santo Domingo has recently designated its commercial area for no further growth because of environmental concerns and strong lobbying from neighborhood groups. Industry and small business are being developed outside city limits on the northern and southern borders.

Option 3, renovating existing space and expanding hours of operation was aggressively pursued, but major asbestos problems were discovered in the main building targeted for renovation. Additionally, the health maintenance organization's labor unions forcibly resisted the notion of expanded hours and threatened an areawide strike. Senior management decided to defer expansion of hours until such actions could be implemented areawide. Thus, Dr. Gallstone was faced with only two options:

- Build new office space on campus
- Develop office space in the emerging population center (approximately 15 miles away).

Table 3. Staff Evaluation of Options 1 Through 4

	1	2	3	4
Net present value (combined capital and operating cost)	$ 5.8 M	$ 5.0 M	$ 6.0 M	$ 6.2 M
Member convenience	M	M	L	H
Membership stimulus	L	L	L	H
Professional staff satisfaction	H	M	H	L
Quality of care	M	M	M	M
Flexibility for future growth	M	M	L	H

*Key: L-Low; M-Medium; H-High

Questions for Discussion

1. Knowing that the medical staff at Santo Domingo prefer on-site expansion and that members of the HMO would prefer the convenience of closer-to-home services in a smaller, less complex setting, how would you go about structuring further analysis and evaluation of the remaining two options?

2. What advice might you offer to Dr. Gallstone in managing his medical staff's expectations?

3. How might he get a favorable decision from the facilities planning committee?

CASE 28

The Creation of a Coordinated Ambulatory Care System

by Robert L. Slaton

For many years, the county board of health operated General Hospital, a public facility that provided medical care to the indigent and an outpatient teaching environment for the school of medicine (SOM) of a major U.S. university. By the late 1950s, the antiquated General Hospital had become inadequate and was scheduled to be replaced. The university agreed to construct a modern teaching hospital to replace it. The new facility was to have an adjacent ambulatory care building (ACB).

While the new facility was being constructed, responsibility for operation of the hospital was transferred to the university. Under university management, the hospital experienced a financial crisis. In response to a large deficit, the university contracted with a management company to operate the new facility, including the outpatient teaching clinics in the ACB.

The management company discontinued the clinics to eliminate the deficit. Clinical departments of the SOM started operating the clinics under a variety of arrangements; some operated their clinics as part of their academic departments, while others created nonprofit foundations or professional service corporations to operate their clinics. The operations became totally separate, with each entity renting space in the ACB.

In 1983, the hospital was leased to a for-profit health care provider. Responsibility for the clinics remained with the respective SOM departments, under the existing arrangements. The clinics were operated independently and without any coordinating mechanism. The clinics developed separate medical records, separate appointment and registration processes, and separate billing systems. There was no system to track patients between clinics, no documentation of the total number of patient visits, and no orderly referral process.

Decision

It was recognized almost immediately that better coordination was needed in order to provide the best possible teaching clinics for the SOM. However, other problems and priorities resulted in no significant action until 1988. At that time, the dean of the SOM, who also served as the university's vice president for hospital affairs, started the process of review to determine what, if any, action should be taken.

Maintaining the status quo was not considered a viable option. Elements of the community were expressing criticism of the outpatient clinics. With separate systems at each clinic, patients were having to provide the same information to the staff at each clinic they visited. Separate medical records made it difficult for a physician to know what was going on with a patient seen in more than one clinic. It was not possible to document the care that was being provided to the public.

There was a certain amount of resistance on the part of the faculty and employees of some of the clinics simply because change is always threatening. However, the dean spent a number of months talking to the department chairs and key staff about the need to make changes and the need to respond to public criticism.

Consideration was given to merging all of the clinics into one unit. However, some of the clinical departments resisted such a dramatic step. Additionally, there was concern about the cost of the renovations that would be required to combine functions that had grown separately for eight years, and the cost of obtaining a centralized management information system.

In 1988, the dean decided to employ someone experienced in government programs and clinic management to develop a plan for achieving greater coordination. The dean requested a new position of associate vice president for hospital affairs — ambulatory care. The person recruited to fill the position was to be responsible for coordinating the SOM ambulatory care activity. The job description of the associate vice president (AVP) included the following responsibilities:

- Develop, implement, and manage an ambulatory care system for the university's SOM, including a centralized process for patient appointments, registration, billing, and records management
- Work with the board of health in the development of a county network of ambulatory care centers
- Work with the clinical departments to ensure that medical student and resident teaching programs have adequate access to ambulatory care patients.

Implementation

In spite of this very direct language, the dean and the new AVP agreed that a plan to coordinate the efforts of the clinics offered a more practical approach than any effort to "take over the clinics." The AVP suggested a consensus-building approach involving a number of people in each clinic. The dean fully supported this approach. The AVP would spend some time in each clinic to learn exactly what it did and to gain an understanding of the problems it faced. For the first few months, his efforts would focus on developing the relationships that would make a coordinated effort possible.

Just prior to the AVP assuming his new duties, a tragedy occurred that altered these plans and changed his role dramatically. The administrator of the department of family practice (DFP) was critically injured in an automobile accident and died a few days later. It had been expected that the DFP would have a key role in any plans that were developed, since the DFP was the lead department in the university's Primary Care Center, the administrative entity that operated as a service bureau to the clinics. It had been assumed that the AVP would work closely with the administrator of the DFP.

The AVP took over as acting administrator of the DFP. The responsibilities of this position occupied virtually all of his time for six months. Since the administrator's death occurred a few days before the end of the fiscal year, the AVP had to deal with the complicated process of year-end closing in an agency where everything was unfamiliar. The situation was complicated when two key staff members resigned to accept other positions in the university.

However, the time the AVP spent in the DFP was invaluable as it offered a crash course in managing the business affairs of the university's teaching clinics. It also offered him the opportunity to become acquainted with other unit business managers as a peer. Any perceived threats were quickly put aside as the other business managers came forward to offer counsel and support.

After a few months, the AVP recruited an assistant who took over the day-to-day operations of the DFP. After six months on the job, she was named department administrator, and the AVP was free to begin implementation of the coordination process envisioned earlier. Implementation had three major steps.

Step 1. Establishing the Advisory Committee and Task Forces

The first step in developing a global system of coordination among all the teaching clinics was the establishment of the ambulatory care system advisory committee. This committee consisted of the chairs (or their designees) of the clinical departments in the SOM. The purpose of the committee was to provide direction in the establishment of a coordinated ambulatory care system. The AVP chaired the 15-member committee, and it began to meet monthly. The establishment of the committee was well received by the department chairs and their unit business managers. Attendance has been excellent and participation active.

The first activity of the committee was to develop a monthly report on the number of patient visits to the clinics by payer source. Since each clinic's data system was different, some time was spent on developing common definitions of payer categories and methodology for counting visits. (Some clinics counted each procedure as a visit while others counted no more than one visit per day per patient.) The committee members all agreed that some composite report was in the interest of the SOM and their respective clinics. After two meetings, a list of payer categories and a counting methodology were made final, and monthly reports were generated.

As soon as the composite reports were available, they were shared with the dean, all department chairs and the board of health. There was general surprise at the number of patients being seen (approximately 150,000 per year) and at the payer mix. The number of Medicaid visits (40 percent) and self-pay or no-insurance visits (30 percent) refuted the criticism that the SOM was not meeting its responsibility to provide care to the area's underserved population.

The second effort of the committee was to establish three special-purpose, short-term task forces made up of appropriate representatives of each clinic to work on improving operation in appointments and registration, billing, and medical records. An outside consultant was hired to serve as a facilitator for the task forces. The members of each task force quickly realized they were all working on the same problem and addressed their tasks with enthusiasm. By pooling their resources and working together, they realized they could achieve more. The task forces met weekly and prepared recommendations to the committee. The task forces defined the following goals:

- To establish a systemwide quality assurance system and identify potential problems to be corrected
- To create a unified ambulatory care database that would allow research in medical outcomes
- To establish a coordinated but decentralized appointment and referral system
- To coordinate medical records and enable physicians to have access to all medical records for an individual patient
- To utilize one sliding-scale fee system and one collection policy to ensure that patients receive the same message from all departments of the SOM.

The task forces continue to work short-term and long-term to implement the objectives designed to meet these goals.

Step 2. Expanding the Primary Care Center

Primary care is a licensure category for a provider of integrated outpatient care. The university held a primary care license for the entire ACB for a number of years. Because of the fragmentation, however, the full implementation of the Primary Care Center had been delayed. Only the departments of family practice and neurology were included in the Primary Care Center. The actual management of the center was handled by the DFP.

It was decided to develop the Primary Care Center as the entity to coordinate the management of additional teaching clinics and to coordinate the effort of all clinics. A two-step process occurred. Management responsibility for the Primary Care Center was transferred from the DFP to the office of the vice president for hospital affairs and the associate vice president for hospital affairs-ambulatory care. The second step was the inclusion of additional clinics in the Primary Care Center: internal medicine, obstetrics/gynecology, ophthalmology, and psychiatry. The Primary Care Center is now a separate department charged with the coordination of selected teaching clinics.

Step 3. Developing a Five-Year Plan

The AVP developed a five-year plan for coordinating all ambulatory care for the SOM's ambulatory care system (see Table 1). In addition to the establishment of the ambulatory care system advisory committee and the three task forces and the identification of the Primary Care Center as the vehicle for coordination of ambulatory care, the five-year plan included the coordination of other clinics, the development of an overall plan for an ambulatory care information system, the creation of a nonprofit foundation board to operate the Primary Care Center, the provision of billing and management services for hospital-based departments, and the formalization of management of the ACB.

Significance of Outcomes

One of the major outcomes of this project was the development of appreciation for the magnitude of the activities of the SOM teaching clinic. The dean and the department chairs were all surprised when the first composite report was developed, indicating the significant number of patient visits occurring annually at the clinics. Almost immediately, a feeling of defensiveness vanished, and a feeling of pride in the amount of work being performed became evident. Moreover, the percentage of the patients who were either indigent or recipients of medical assistance showed a significant commitment to taking care of the less fortunate in the community.

Major attention was focused on the teaching clinics for the first time in a number of years. The department chairs became much more involved and aware of what was going on in their clinics. The dean and the department chairs committed additional resources for improving the clinics. The involvement of administrative staff, physicians, the advisory committee, and the three task

Table 1. Five-Year Plan for Full Implementation of the Unified Ambulatory Care System

	1990	1991	1992	1993	1994
Establish the advisory committee	■				
Establish the Primary Care Center as a separate department	■	■			
Initiate Primary Care task force	■	■			
1. Appointments/registration	■				
2. Billing	■				
3. Medial records	■				
4. Laboratory	■				
5. Medical directors	■				
6. Directors of nursing	■				
Incorporate additional clinics	■	■			
Ophthalmology	■				
Obstetrics/gynecology	■				
Psychiatry	■				
Internal medicine		■			
Pediatrics — Infants		■			
Pediatrics — Children & Youth		■			
Coordinate specialty clinics				■	
Surgery				■	
Orthopedic surgery				■	
Install ambulatory care information system	■	■	■	■	■
Develop and issue request for proposal		■			
Appointments/registration		■			
Billing		■			
Medical records		■			
Quality control			■		
Research				■	■
Create nonprofit foundation to operate primary care center		■	■		
Complete legal research		■	■		
Implement nonprofit foundation			■		
Offer billing/management for hospital-based services				■	
Anesthesiology				■	
Emergency medicine				■	
Pathology				■	
Radiology				■	
Formalize management of ambulatory care system		■	■		
Ambulatory care building		■			
Other university ambulatory care locations		■			
Nonuniversity ambulatory care locations		■			

forces led to significant consensus building and involvement in finding solutions to serious problems.

Lessons Learned

Major problems were identified and are currently being addressed.

Quality Assurance

Employees expressed concerns about quality of care due to, but not limited to, the inability to obtain medical records from other clinics, inability to see the growing number of patients who request medical care, lack of coordination among the clinics in referrals, and appointment clerks being required to do triage.

Inability to Meet the Demand for Medical Services

Six of the eight clinics indicated that they could not see on a timely basis new patients who were referred to them from other clinics or who request services on their own, and that they sometimes have trouble seeing on a timely basis current patients who request additional or follow-up medical services.

Database and Research

Members of the medical records task force suggested that each clinic could export data into a common data base for ambulatory care research. There is no good way to do research on ambulatory care in the absence of a common database. The SOM would not be able to stay in the mainstream of research and teaching without such a database.

Liability

Professional and support staff identified six specific concerns about potential liability.

Fees

The clinics were losing hundreds of thousands of dollars annually in fees because of their inability to see a larger number of patients. Among the constraints were nonclinical functions occupying clinical space. A number of examination rooms could be freed by moving nonclinical functions to other locations. Furthermore, some physicians in some clinics did not sign the paperwork required to receive Medicare reimbursement.

Postscript

In the five years following this effort, the SOM was able to make many changes through consensus building. These changes have worked for the betterment of the system and patient care. On the other hand, the five-year plan achieved only about half of what it hoped to achieve.

A number of events interfered along the way with the achievement of some goals and caused the modification of other goals. These include:

- A fairly divisive two-year process to change the faculty practice plan
- A protracted and divisive debate about health care reform legislation at the state level
- Two changes of ownership of the company managing the hospital.

The remaining goals — creating a nonprofit foundation to operate the Primary Care Center, formalizing management of the ambulatory care system, and creating a unified information system — are being pursued very aggressively as the SOM tries to position the clinics to provide Medicaid managed care.

Questions for Discussion

1. If you were the associate vice president, would you have approached the task of consolidating the clinics any differently? If so, how?

2. Would you have designed the job description of the Associate Vice President differently? If so, how?

3. How will you know when the project has been successful? What measures will you use?

4. What were several of the key organizational elements that needed to be in place before the associate vice president could move the project forward?

5. Why was there resistance to centralization from some of the clinics? How could this resistance have been defused in a more timely manner?

PART V

Short Interactive
Case Studies

Decision-Making Time

by Austin Ross

You are the CEO. Your chief operating officer, Jeff, has been in that position and under your direction for the last 15 years. While things seemed to be working before, you are now receiving a continual stream of information that this individual is no longer performing effectively. He is well liked, but the respect of those who report to him has diminished because he has grown "out of touch with what is going on."

Jeff has consistently demonstrated loyalty, typically works a ten-hour day, and believes that he is doing a good job.

As you begin to study the situation, you discover what you have suspected for some time, that he lacks a management style that is compatible with the "new breed" of managers. He lacks strategic sensitivity. You also recognize that you have been procrastinating. You have not been conveying honest feedback to Jeff at the annual review time or at other times.

The recent and unexpected announcement of the resignation of both your planning director and the chief financial officer comes at a bad time. Both were important to the organization. In exit interviews, both indicated that a major reason for relocating was their inability to communicate with Jeff.

You also suddenly realize that your inability to do something about the situation may be eroding your personal credibility. After very careful and thoughtful reflection, you decide that action must be taken and soon.

Questions for Discussion

1. What action should you take, and how?
2. What could you have done earlier?
3. What will happen if you continue to procrastinate?
4. What management concepts have been violated in this case?

The Case of the Accidental Encounter

by Austin Ross

You are the president of the board of Everlasting Memorial Hospital in suburban Walnut City. You are enjoying a nonalcoholic beverage after 18 holes of golf, and you engage in a conversation with the president of the board of Granitesville Memorial, your primary competitor. You know each other socially. You are a 10 handicap, while she is a 12.

You are well aware that, all over the United States, hospitals are clumping together and merging or creating alliances. So far, for 15 years, Everlasting has been highly competitive with Granitesville. In fact, you don't really trust those folks at all — and yet? It is your understanding that there haven't been any serious discussions about linking with Granitesville, even though this might be a good strategy to protect your market from those urban centers that are beginning to buy up the territory. (At least, this is what you have heard from your hospital CEO.)

After half an hour of conversation on this hot day, you wonder whether it would be appropriate to raise a simple question with your competitor's board president. Finally, you blurt, "Do you ever think that it might be possible for our two hospitals to really talk about health care? Maybe we aren't doing as well as we should for our respective communities by competing so aggressively?"

You expect a cool response. Instead, you are stunned to hear that your colleague has been thinking the same thing. She responds by saying, "Maybe we should act more on behalf of the community and be less interested in protecting our own turf."

You both decide at that instant that this represents a unique opportunity. Right there at the golf club, you mutually decide to develop an agenda for a high-level meeting about the issues that might be raised. Fortunately, both of you are equipped with the stub pencils you used to record your golfing scores. You grab some napkins and start designing the agenda.

Question for Discussion

- What issues or questions would you record that might be included on the initial board agenda for discussion? (Limit the agenda to six items.)

Consulting 101

by Austin Ross

Part I

You are a prominent consultant specializing in strategic planning and organizational development. Your clients are primarily health care providers, but you have dabbled a bit in the airline and savings and loan industries as well.

Last week you received a call from the executive director of the state hospital association. He indicated he would like to meet with you, and you mutually agreed to meet in his office. Other then setting up the meeting, he gave you no clues about what the meeting would be about.

Question for Discussion

- What, if anything, would you do to prepare for the meeting?

Part II

The day of the meeting has arrived, and you enter his office. The executive director is there, and he has also arranged for the associate director of the association to attend.

Question for Discussion

- Two of you will serve as the association's executive director and associate director. Two of you will serve as the consultant. The rest of the class will be there to back you up. You may use them as you see fit, but only the two designated consultants can interact with the executive director and associate director. Please proceed now with the meeting.

Media Mania

by Austin Ross

You are the administrator of Small Town Medical Group Practice. The phone rings, and it is Tanya Tauker, editor of the local news page of the *Small Town Times*, your local newspaper. Tanya has heard word of a potential affiliation between your medical group practice and Sunnyside Medical Center, the local hospital. You are caught off guard, because these discussions have been quite confidential up until now.

Only last night, there was a secret meeting between members of the executive committee of Sunnyside's board of directors and key physicians from the group practice. The meeting was a bit acrimonious, with the physicians accusing the hospital officials of realizing substantial financial gains based on referrals made by the group practice. The physician owners of the group practice feel the profits have not been fairly divided, and future control of patient revenues is a major sticking point to the ongoing discussions about a proposed physician-hospital venture.

Tanya makes several provocative comments, alluding to the hot rhetoric that went on during the meeting. You begin to suspect that there may be an inside leak to the newspaper. You're not sure who might have done this, or what the purpose might be.

Question for Discussion
- What will you do?

Team Trauma

by Mary Richardson

You are newly hired as the assistant administrator for a multispecialty group practice. The practice is well established and noted for its community spirit and sensitivity toward meeting community needs. The practice includes three very busy and successful perinatologists. The perinatologists are quite concerned about the number of infants they are delivering who are at high risk for subsequent developmental problems because of their prematurity. Often, these infants spend weeks and even months in a special care nursery, and then are released with little or no follow-up care. In an effort to provide appropriate follow-up, physicians within the practice are experimenting with an interdisciplinary team concept. This concept is supposed to offer developmental follow-up assessments at periodic intervals and provide consultation to other providers who may also be involved in the care of these children after they leave the hospital.

The team has been operational for six months, and the administrator has identified some problems. First of all, the perinatologist who organized the team is a bit autocratic in running it and has angered the two nurse practitioners who participate with the team by behaving in a condescending manner toward them. Second, it was suggested that a developmental psychologist be enlisted, perhaps from among the private practitioner community, in order to provide developmental assessments. However, the perinatologist feels quite capable of making those assessments based on the physical evaluation conducted during each visit. Finally, the administrator has strong suspicions that this whole team idea is costing more money than it is generating in revenues.

Question for Discussion

- What's your plan?

Midtown Community Home Health Center

by Mary Richardson

You are the director of Midtown Community Home Health Center. Your center has been in operation for more than 15 years, providing home health services to older adults and persons with disabilities, including people with both physical and cognitive impairments. Generally, your revenue source has been out-of-pocket payment by clients (20 percent), Medicaid (40 percent), grants (20 percent), and Medicare (20 percent). Home health care has typically been considered a community or public health care service, since it is financed largely through governmental or public mechanisms. Many of the services are to populations that are not covered by regular health insurance, or that may have some coverage but not for home care.

Your state has formed a commission to study health care reform initiatives, because of the growing concern over the number of people who are without any insurance, and because Medicaid is becoming a significant portion of the state budget. As a result of the high probability of reform legislation coming about because of the work of this commission and the strong political support for change statewide, many of the larger health care systems are beginning to expand into primary and community-based care. They are using a number of different approaches, including developing their own clinics, affiliating with existing group practices and purchasing smaller hospitals and incorporating their primary care services into the larger system — just to name a few.

Home health care has not been a major player when discussions of health care reform have taken place. In fact, it is not entirely clear where home health will ultimately fit in, although it seems that caring for persons in the home — or at least in the community rather than in an expensive inpatient facility — will have great appeal under reforms that seek lower-cost solutions to health care delivery.

As director of Midtown Community Home Health Care, you have been approached by senior managers from the six major health care systems that serve your community. They are anxious to talk to you about merging, although the discussions have not gone far enough to determine what that really means. You have strong referral relationships with two of them. In fact, your referrals have primarily come from hospital discharge planners. Physicians are also a referral base, but not nearly so significant as hospitals.

You are getting ready to make a presentation to your board of directors, composed of a physician from one of the systems; an administrator from a smaller community hospital that also provides a lot of referrals; and an accountant, a lawyer, and a business owner from the community. The board members haven't spent much time talking about health care reform, so you're not sure how knowledgeable they are concerning the issues at stake. You need to give them an overview of the situation, along with some recommendations about how to analyze this situation, and come up with some criteria for deciding what to do.

Question for Discussion

- Describe, in four pages or less, what you will say to your board.

Physicians as Managers

by Mary Richardson

You are an internist working within an integrated network of three hospitals and seven clinic sites. As a result of plans for expansion, there is a move afoot to expand the primary care network substantially, while reducing the number of subspecialty practitioners within the system. You have been quite involved in medical staff management, serving on committees and task forces struggling with the many complex issues facing the system. You are still quite active in your practice, and there is an expectation that your clinical productivity should remain fairly high. Yet, because you have good conceptual and planning skills and you hold considerable influence with other physicians in the system, there seems to be a growing, almost unmanageable, demand for your time in the strategic decision-making committees that seem to pop up regularly. You are particularly in demand when it comes to developing strategies for changing physician roles or the specialty mix within the system. You are reluctant to limit your participation in these important committees because the decisions that are made have the potential for substantial effect on your colleagues and, ultimately, on clinical practice. Moreover, you are enjoying this expanded role. However, management within the system doesn't seem to be embracing physicians as a part of the formal management structure as new plans and organizational changes go forward. This seems like an oversight from your perspective. You are thinking about approaching the senior management team with a proposal for including physicians in management on a more formal basis.

Question for Discussion
- What are the elements of your argument?

The Leader's Mantle

by Austin Ross

Rick is a very successful manager of a large multispecialty clinic. He is so successful that his time is much in demand, and he hires an assistant. Joan is highly intelligent and arrives with impeccable credentials. She proves to be most capable. Over a six-month period, Rick's dependence on her increases continuously. She handles appointment schedules with dispatch and gradually becomes so efficient that she asks for and receives additional help in the form of a front-line secretary to work for her.

Rick has heard some rumbles about people having trouble getting to see him, but he discounts this as a sign that he is simply much in demand. What he doesn't know is that increasing numbers of the clinic staff suspect that he has been "captured" by Joan, who is running roughshod over employees and outsiders whom she views as unimportant interruptions in Rick's busy schedule. (Joan is very careful to take good care of those who are influential in the clinic and to Rick.) Insiders have become fearful of her because of her influence over Rick.

The problem starts to surface when a well-respected colleague comments to Rick on how inaccessible Rick has become and, further, that a number of Rick's colleagues now perceive him to be on an ego trip. Rick decides he needs to check out the rumors of his unavailability and finds to his amazement that indeed a number of his close colleagues in the field have backed away from him because they can never get their calls returned. They had concluded that Rick, smart as he is, wouldn't make himself inaccessible unless he wanted to be inaccessible.

Questions for Discussion

1. What are the base problems that contributed to Rick's dilemma?
2. How could he have prevented this from happening?
3. Is this an unusual circumstance? If so, why?

Tantrum Time

by Austin Ross

You are the clinic manager. One of your prominent surgeons, Dr. Flexner, has a bad temper. Lately, he has been verbally abusing several of his office assistants and, in particular, has been picking on Sally. This morning, one of the clinic's most loyal patients drops by your office and hesitantly asks to have her care transferred to another physician because of the way Dr. Flexner always shouts at Sally.

Question for Discussion

- How would you handle this situation?

The Value of Your Word

by Austin Ross

After months of effort, you and the chief financial officer have finally negoti-ated a reasonable specialty service contract with a regional HMO, and it has received voice approval from the officers of your executive committee, who have been kept well informed throughout the entire process. You meet with the CEO of the health maintenance organization, and you notify her that the transaction has been approved subject to the formality of a vote of the board. The vote of the clinic's board is to take place next week, and you decide to take a few days of vacation before the board meeting.

When you return, you are astounded to find that in your absence an influ-ential clinic primary care physician has lobbied the board, and the board chair has authorized a telephone vote on the proposal. The board voted 6-to-3 to reject the arrangement. When you convey this news to the HMO's CEO, she comes unglued, because her board has acted favorably, based on your word. She tells you that she will now do everything within her means to keep any and all of the HMO's business away from your clinic. You have never been threatened in that fashion before. In fact, you are totally dismayed with the whole process and spend considerable time reflecting on why this happened and how it happened without your involvement.

Questions for Discussion

1. What conclusions did you reach after reflecting on those two points?
2. Are there other questions that you should be pondering? If so, what are they?

Twenty-first Century Diagnostic Center

by Margaret McDonald and Lynn Zimmerman

Part I

At the Twenty-first Century Diagnostic Center, it was becoming widely known that patients were not happy about how or when they were notified of test and procedure results. It seemed to you, one of four section managers, that you were hearing a growing number of referring physicians and office staff complain about the number of inquiries about their patients' test results. Sometimes it was just a request for additional interpretation of the result or direction on what to do next, but most often patients commented on how long the time had been since the test and wondered if the result could have been lost. Most of your staff are reporting rumors of physicians grumbling about sending their patients to the other center in town.

Currently, however, the center has more demand than it can currently handle and is planning a major expansion. Between the increasing patient volume and planning for the new building, your people feel overworked just managing day-to-day.

You believe though, that over time, dissatisfied patients and physicians will only hurt the center, and something needs to be done.

Question for Discussion

- What steps would you take to begin to tackle this problem?

Part II

When you talked with the other three section managers, only one seemed interested in doing something about the high level of dissatisfaction. The other two felt there would be no noticeable organizational effects, so the other more pressing issues were their priority. However, one of these sections had an employee who voiced an interest in being a part of the work group — a new employee who thought participation might be educational.

You assemble a small work group, the assessment team, which included people from the two receptive sections, and the interested employee of the third group. This small work group identified the current process and brainstormed possible problem areas. An outside firm gathered survey data. The results were astounding.

- Of the patients who had received a test over the last month, 55 percent stated the reporting practices were poor.

- Sixty percent said that, if they had a choice in the future, they would go to a different center for tests.

- Of all referring physicians over the last month, 70 percent stated they were seriously considering referring patients to another laboratory for most routine tests.

Many of the detailed survey questions reflected a similar level of dissatisfaction. There were, however, some key points that seemed to drive the overall dissatisfaction that patients experienced. These were: (1) an initial understanding of how and when the test result would be reported, (2) a longer-than-expected wait time for result, and (3) poor explanation of the result when it was received. The physicians' dissatisfaction was driven primarily by the patients' dissatisfaction and the additional work that generated for their offices.

Questions for Discussion

1. How would you move forward with the change process?
2. Whom would you involve, and why?

Part III

Congratulations! The evaluation is back, and it is clear that the new process does in fact improve patient and provider satisfaction substantially. Your long, hard work has paid off, at least for the patients who went through your section and were sent by physicians who participated in the testing of the new process. This group reported:

- Only 6 percent of the patients who received a test stated the result reporting practices were poor.

- Only 3 percent said that, if they had a choice, they would go to a different center.

- Eighty-five percent of the referring physicians who participated said the process for reporting test results was excellent.

No changes were seen in other physicians' patients, who were seen in the other three sections. Upon hearing results, the second invested team is eager to implement the change. However, the planning efforts for the expansion are intensifying, and your boss does not seem to be supporting the efforts of the second section in making the change. It seems she hasn't had time for this project lately — or for you, for that matter. It has been difficult to pin her down regarding resources and timing for the second implementation. The other two sections are not interested in changing their practices, even with compelling data to support the worthiness of the effort. They believe that, since they are the two departments that do more specialized testing and the results often take a longer time to report, the same results would not be seen in their patients and consequently their physicians. They also found out that the information system was not designed to support their unique data needs.

Your boss says she is pleased with the results in your section, but her actions are not supporting her words in implementing the changes further. You're wondering if she might be threatened by the change or possibly the success of the project? In any case, she is acting very strangely. You are about ready to quit, or go back to your own section and "just do your job," frustrated that all your work will go no further.

Question for Discussion

- What could have happened differently, and how?

.

New on the Job

by Margaret McDonald and Lynn Zimmerman

This is it, the day of the big presentation, your first presentation to the Mercy Hospital administrative team, of which your boss, Joan, is a regular member. All of the activities of your first three months on the job have led up to this meeting. Most of the members you will be meeting for the first time, and you know it's critical to make a good impression. You will be presenting the Employee Morale Survey, a survey of employees to assess many aspects of their working environment and attitudes. The development of this survey has taken all of your time since you started in the personnel department.

During the first week of your job, your boss reviewed this initial work assignment and its relationship to some of the recent changes within the hospital. You also attended the organizational orientation for new employees. This provided you with some valuable information about organization policies and expectations. Like many hospitals across the nation, Mercy is experiencing a decline in census and has been forced to reduce staffing levels in nursing as well as in the supporting ancillary departments. Of the staff who have stayed with the hospital, many have had to change their work schedules to accommodate patient needs. The last year has been a stressful period for everyone at Mercy.

All of the uncertainty and change, Joan explained, has resulted in the department heads throughout the hospital, and employees, complaining much more than they used to. A couple of the frequent comments were that Mercy didn't have the feeling of family it used to have, and it wasn't a place that cared about its employees — it just cared about profit. Joan thought it would be a good idea to test these impressions, to determine the actual level of employee satisfaction or dissatisfaction, and then to provide the department heads with information to assist them in their planning efforts.

Eager to make a good impression, you dove into the assignment, focusing your work on this high-priority and visible project. You spent considerable time researching the literature and checking current textbooks on survey design. You even contacted the university and consulted research experts to design a technically perfect survey instrument that included all of the commonly asked questions. You are confident that you have a superb survey tool.

And now it's time for the presentation. It consists of an introduction of the topic by your boss, discussing the perceived effects of the experiences from the past year, and the need to substantiate these effects before beginning programs to improve morale. Next, Joan introduces you, the newest member of the personnel department, as the manager of this important project. You seize your opportunity and explain the design of the survey, the information that will be produced from the data, the timeline, level of individual involvement needed, and projected costs associated with survey — all of which have been carefully thought through and written up. You then offer a period of time for questions and general discussion.

You are devastated. No one seems to think the survey is worthwhile. You are bewildered. It seems obvious to you that this is necessary information. Some of the members claim the questions to be asked would be meaningless: the words are wrong, the employees wouldn't be honest, and the information would be flawed. Many felt they already knew how their employees felt and didn't need a survey, and some thought the information would be better if each supervisor sat and talked with staff specifically about these issues. The general opinion was, it flopped ten years ago, it will flop again.

Question for Discussion

- What could have been done to prevent or to prepare for the resistance to the survey?

Storming Norms

by Margaret McDonald and Lynn Zimmerman

You are an associate administrator at Everglade Memorial Hospital, one of seven midsize hospitals in the ChampionCare Health System. You have been assigned by your boss, who got the assignment from the corporate operations chief, to lead a highly visible and strategically important quality improvement project. A recent patient survey indicated that a majority of patients feel a high level of frustration with how complaints are handled at the hospital. Your job is to come up with a simple and responsive complaint-handling process. Your hospital will serve as pilot site and, after an evaluation, the plan is for the improved process to be adopted systemwide.

Having recently attended a total quality management training program, you feel you are well prepared for the task, and you are excited by the challenge. You know that your first step is to assemble a team that represents the multiple stakeholders affected by this process. After asking various department heads around the hospital to suggest potential members, and after talking with those individuals, you have an eager quality improvement team. The team consists of a hospital admitting manager, the pharmacy manager, the head nurse of 4-West, a gastroenterologist, a radiology technician, and a nurse's aide.

At your first meeting, you decide the first task at hand is to define team norms and responsibilities. Together, the team commits to the following:

1. Arrive on time.

2. Read materials and do assignments prior to the meeting.

3. Share information and solicit comments about the quality improvement project with people in their functional areas.

4. Be able to represent genuinely or speak on behalf of their functional areas during discussions.

5. Air opinions about a decision prior to the decision being made. Once a decision is made by the group, take ownership and responsibility for it.

This meeting, and the next one, ended on a positive note. The team was off to a great start and determined to do well in the data-gathering phase of the project. One minor irritation was Dr. Guts's tardiness for the two meetings. He was very apologetic, and he had good reasons for being late, but the team was visibly annoyed. You decide to let it go and hope that Dr. Guts would read the team's signals and shape up. It turned out to be a good strategy.

In the design phase of the project, things got more challenging. There were decidedly different opinions about how to design an effective complaint-handling process. Most team members wanted a decentralized process that allowed the person who received the complaint to address it. However, the head nurse, Ms. Adams, resolutely advocated for a hospital ombudsperson to address patient complaints. "Nurses are too busy to handle every little patient problem."

After a lengthy discussion, the team decided to design a decentralized complaint-handling process. In the end, Ms. Adams conceded to the logic of this approach as a better way to meet patients' needs.

After that meeting, progress went downhill. It seems Ms. Adams reported at the weekly head nurse meeting that the quality improvement team wasn't taking into account nurses' needs, and she subtly counseled the nurses to sabotage the effort.

You hear about this at a dinner party from another head nurse who is also a guest. She also tells you that the meeting was the first time the nurses had formally heard about the quality improvement project from Ms. Adams. Furthermore, she tells you that Ms. Adams doesn't have much credibility with some of the nurses.

Steam is coming out of your ears. Good thing it's Saturday night and you have time to cool off on Sunday before you have to chair your next team meeting at seven o'clock Monday morning.

Questions for Discussion

1. What do you do?
2. What could you have done to avoid this problem in the first place?

Family Care Medical Group

by Margaret McDonald and Lynn Zimmerman

Allison Jones is the founder of Family Care Medical Group. In the middle 1960s, after the implementation of Medicaid and Medicare, Dr. Jones decided that hooking up with some other physicians would be a good idea. She thought that sharing practice overhead, such as the administrative costs associated with patient appointment and billing systems, which she thought might increase with the onset of Medicaid and Medicare; sharing building overhead; and sharing nursing costs would be a more efficient way to use those services, minimize those costs, and maximize her income. Over time, she has shared these expenses with several family practice physicians. The working agreement is that the physicians share these costs in proportion to how much time they spend in the office and by volume of patient visits. Additionally, they have committed to share the hospital call schedule. The physicians maintain their independent practices and receive the revenue brought in by their particular group of patients.

Today, Family Care Medical Group is a medical group practice consisting of four family practice physicians and their support staff, located in Suburbia. Patients visiting the clinic range from young working families to elderly patients who have retired in Suburbia. Chris Eager, the clinic manager for the last six months, has noticed an increasing number of patients requesting same-day appointments for urgent health care needs. They don't expect urgent appointment slots on Saturdays yet. At the same time, these patients also want the clinic to make available noon and evening appointment times. Generally, seniors want to be able to schedule regular appointments in advance. More customers are complaining about not being able to get scheduled visits, but there is also more demand for urgent visits. For the record, most patients want to see their own doctor and want quick visits. That is, they don't want to wait too long, and when they get in to see their physician, they want to have the time to establish a bond and ask questions.

In mulling over an approach to handle these complaints, Ms. Eager takes stock of the current situation.

Dr. Jones

Dr. Jones, the practice matriarch, has been practicing family medicine for almost 30 years. Her patients are predominantly elderly and have grown up with her as their family physician. Dr. Jones is happily awaiting retirement and has adjusted her schedule accordingly. Her typical day starts at 9:00 A.M. with her hospital rounds for about an hour (most physicians round from 7:30 A.M. to 9:00 A.M.), and her last patient appointment is at 2:45 P.M. On nice Fridays (and, more recently, any nice day), she'll often skip out for a couple sets of tennis, which requires some creative juggling of her appointments at the last minute. Dr. Jones doesn't see a problem regarding her routine. According to her, her patients go with the flow and don't demand too much.

Dr. Bright

Dr. Bright is the newest addition to the Family Care Medical Group. Chief resident of the family practice residency at the University of Hawaii, Dr. Bright joined Family Care Medical Group two years ago right out of residency. He practices both pediatrics and obstetrics/gynecology. He is definitely a physician of the '90s — extremely energetic and dedicated to serving his patients' needs yet committed to balancing his work life with his personal life. Being the new kid on the block, he typically gets the new patients, usually with the most health care needs. His patients are mostly young professional working families with young children or single working professionals. This population has a high need for convenience and urgent care appointments. Because Dr. Bright delivers babies, he is often at the hospital overnight, which causes his day schedule to be sporadic and unpredictable. When Dr. Bright is in the office, he adamantly protects his lunch hour for a five-mile run. He then drives to the hospital, where he showers and does his daily rounding.

Dr. Stable

Dr. Stable has been with Family Care Medical Group for 12 years. She has a stable, evenly mixed patient panel and takes on new patients fairly regularly. She likes her set routine: rounding first thing in the morning and seeing patients in the clinic until about 5:00 P.M. She and her husband have patterned their life together and enjoy spending time with their two high-school–age kids. Dr. Stable likes things just the way they are.

Dr. Dogood

Dr. Dogood practices half-time at the clinic and has been doing so for about five years. In his other life, he practices half-time at an inner-city community clinic. After his residency at Cook County Hospital in Chicago, he made a personal commitment to continue to serve the low-income, typically underserved population that presented there. Dr. Dogood's schedule changes on a monthly basis, but rarely changes once it is set.

The Nursing Staff

Three nurses are currently on staff — one full-time and two that job-share. Their workload has been steadily increasing over time. They are providing more direct patient care, as the physicians are becoming less available and asking them to do more. Patients are beginning to ask for appointments with the nurses only. Generally, the nurses are pleased with their higher level of involvement in patient care and decision making but are frustrated with the lack of defined role, which sometimes causes conflict. They are also beginning to ask about higher compensation for their increased responsibilities.

The Office Staff

The office staff is really caught in the middle. The medical receptionist, who is responsible for patient appointments and medical records, is spending more and more of her time moving patients around to accommodate urgent requests and the doctors' schedules. This has become so time-intensive that the billing clerk often has to serve as a backup, answering phones and pulling records. This affects the billing clerk's ability to get the bills out in a timely fashion and post payments as they come in. Both the receptionist and the billing clerk are extremely frustrated at what they see as the doctors' lack of responsiveness to patient needs.

The Big Meeting

Ms. Eager ascertains from all this that the current appointment-making process, or lack of one, is causing unpredictability of patient flow, which is causing inefficient work processes, disgruntled employees, and dissatisfied patients. She decides to test the waters with each of the physicians individually before her regular meeting with all of them next week. This is what she hears.

Dr. Jones says, "Things seem fine to me. I've practiced this way for 30 years, and my patients know me and my habits. Anyway, I'm thinking about tapering off my working hours."

Dr. Bright says, "I'm open to changing my routine when I'm scheduled here, but my family and workout time are important to me. I won't compromise on that. Otherwise, this place will eat me alive."

Dr. Stable says, "I'm willing to listen to my patients and meet their specific needs. I'm not willing to cover to accommodate the whims of my colleagues."

Dr. Dogood says, "The agreement I made when I came on board was that I would be able to maintain my community clinic practice. I'd be willing to change my hours in any way around my community clinic schedule, but I do have to eat and do my laundry!"

Ms. Eager's meeting with the group is tomorrow.

Questions for Discussion

1. What should Ms. Eager do to balance all these needs and move forward?

2. What should her approach be for tomorrow's discussion?

List of Contributors

Ronald M. Andersen, Ph.D., Wasserman Professor and Chair, Program in Health Policy & Management, Department of Health Services, School of Public Health, University of California, Los Angeles

Carl Bellas, Ph.D., Dean, School of Business, Samford University, Birmingham, Alabama

Patty Belson, Special Projects Consultant, Kaiser Permanente, Oakland, California

John C. Blanchard, M.H.A., Student and Research Assistant, Department of Health Services, School of Public Health & Community Medicine, University of Washington, Seattle

Keith Boles, Ph.D., Associate Professor, Health Services Management, University of Missouri, Columbia

Robert Boyle, Jr., Chief Executive Officer, Cardiovascular Provider Resources, LP, Dallas, Texas

Bruce Deal, Ph.D. Candidate in Public Policy, Kennedy School of Government, Harvard University, Cambridge, Massachusetts

D. Cheryl Erins, FACMPE, Practice Administrator, Swedish Covenant Hospital, Chicago, Illinois

Jerome I. Fink, FACMPE, Administrator, Vann-Atlantic Orthopaedic Specialists, PC, Norfolk, Virginia

Steven Paul Fiore, FACMPE, Executive Vice President, Orthopedic Group, Inc., Pawtucket, Rhode Island

Susan Flautt, Eldercare Products Manager, Kaiser Permanente, Oakland, California

Nancy M. Friedrich, FACHE, Senior Management Consultant, Superior Consultant Company, Inc., Bainbridge Island, Washington

Daniel Garson-Angert, Doctoral Candidate, Center for Health Policy Research & Education, School of Health Policy & Administration, University of North Carolina-Chapel Hill

Paul Halverson, Dr.P.H., FACHE, Assistant Professor, Department of Health Policy & Administration, School of Public Health, University of North Carolina-Chapel Hill

Charles E. Hawley, Vice President, Continuum Development and Long Term Care, Sisters of Providence Health System, Seattle, Washington

Diana W. Hilberman, Director of Field Studies, Program in Health Policy & Management, Department of Health Services, School of Public Health, University of California, Los Angeles

Linda Kay Horton, FACMPE, Regional Operations Director, Medalia HealthCare LLC, Seattle, Washington

Christine Hurley, Director, Bailey Boushay House, Seattle, Washington

Arnold D. Kaluzny, Ph.D., Professor, Department of Health Policy & Administration, School of Public Health and Cecil G. Sheps Center for Health Services, University of North Carolina-Chapel Hill

Joel Koemptgen, FACMPE, Vice President of Regional Services, St. Mary's Medical Center, Duluth, Minnesota

W. Paul Kory, M.D., Assistant Professor of Pediatrics & Director of Research, Division of Community Pediatrics, Montefiore Medical Center/Albert Einstein College of Medicine, New York

Therese M. Martaus, Director of Care Management, Group Health Cooperative of Puget Sound-Community Health and Long Term Care, Seattle, Washington

Margaret McDonald, Manager, Department of Project Services, Group Health Cooperative of Puget Sound-Hospital System, Seattle, Washington

Patricia H. Mintz, President, The Healthcare Redesign Group, Alameda, California

Chad L. Peter, FACMPE, Clinic Administrator, Defiance Clinic, Defiance, Ohio

Janet Piehl, Medical Student (M.D. expected June 1996), Mercer Island, Washington

Paul F. Primeau, FACMPE, Vice President, Unified Health Care Network, West Chester, Illinois

Mary Richardson, Ph.D., Professor and Director, Graduate Program in Health Services Administration, Department of Health Services, School of Public Health and Community Medicine, University of Washington, Seattle

Katie Ricklefs, Medical Group Administrator, Vallejo Medical Center, Vallejo, California

Austin Ross, Professor, Graduate Program in Health Services Administration, Department of Health Services, School of Public Health and Community Medicine, University of Washington, Seattle

Mary E. Ryan, FACMPE, Director, Physician Management Services, Intracoastal Health Corporation, West Palm Beach, Florida

Katharine Sacks Sanders, Director, Community Health Networks, Washington Health Foundation, Washington State Hospital Association, Seattle, Washington

Lane Savitch, Administrator, Monroe Valley General, Monroe, Washington

Mark Secord, President, Secord Consulting, Seattle, Washington

Stephanie A. Simon, Administrative Analyst, Group Health Cooperative of Puget Sound, Seattle, Washington

Robert L. Slaton, Ed.D., FACMPE, Associate Vice President of Ambulatory Care, Primary Care Center/Executive Director, School of Medicine, University of Louisville, Kentucky

John F. Tiscornia, Partner, Arthur Andersen LLP, Seattle, Washington

Paul R. Torrens, M.D., Professor, Program in Health Policy & Management, Department of Health Services, School of Public Health, University of California, Los Angeles

Susan Tuller, Manager of Care Systems, Group Health Cooperative of Puget Sound, Kelsey Creek, Washington

Carolyn Watts Madden, Ph.D., Professor, Department of Health Services, School of Public Health & Community Medicine, University of Washington, Seattle

Lynn Zimmerman, Senior Financial & Operations Analyst, Group Health Cooperative of Puget Sound-Office of Practice Analysis, Seattle, Washington

Howard Zuckerman, Ph.D., Professor, School of Health Administration & Policy, Arizona State College of Business, Tempe, Arizona

About the Editors

Austin Ross

Austin Ross is currently a professor in the Department of Health Services at the University of Washington's School of Public Health and Community Medicine. His teaching and research interests focus on integrated health care systems, group practice and ambulatory care, and leadership and management. Austin is also a national consultant for Arthur Andersen and Company (Health Services Division).

In addition, Austin is Vice President and Executive Administrator Emeritus of the Virginia Mason Medical Center in Seattle, Washington. After receiving his master's degree in Public Health from the University of California in Berkeley in 1955, Austin joined Virginia Mason's administrative staff and was with Virginia Mason until his retirement in 1991.

Austin is currently an active member of numerous national organizations. He is a past chairman of the American College of Healthcare Executives, and past president of the National Medical Group Management Association, the Association of Western Hospitals (Healthcare Forum), the Washington State Hospital Association, and other health service and community organizations. In addition he has served as a project consultant to the Robert Wood Johnson Foundation and the W. K. Kellogg Foundation.

Over his professional career, Austin has been the recipient of several awards including the Gold Medal from the American College of Healthcare Executives, the Harry J. Harwick Award from the American College of Medical Group Administrators, and the Executive Administrator of the Year Award from the American Group Practice Association.

Austin is also the author and coauthor of several books and has published over 50 articles with a special focus on management and strategic planning. Austin's latest book, *Cornerstones of Leadership for Health Services Executives,* was published by Health Administration Press and awarded the 1993 James A. Hamilton Book of the Year Award by the American College of Healthcare Executives.

Mary Richardson

Mary Richardson is currently the Director for the Graduate Program in Health Services Administration; an associate professor for the Department of Health Services, School of Public Health and Community Medicine; Co-Director for the Center for Disability Policy and Research; and Discipline Head for the Discipline Health Administration of the Child Development and Mental Retardation Center, all at the University of Washington.

Currently, Dr. Richardson is studying health promotion and health management for persons with disabilities and chronic conditions. Based on previous research, she reported on the integration of health and social services for persons with disabilities through interagency coordination, developing model approaches and documenting successful statewide efforts. She completed a Joseph P. Kennedy, Jr. Fellowship in Public Policy (1989–90) working for Senator Tom Harkin on the Subcommittee on Disability Policy. In 1993 she became a Policy Fellow for the Packard Roundtable for Children.

Dr. Richardson is active on a number of boards, including the editorial board of the *Journal of Health Administration Education*, the AUPHA Board of Directors (Chair-Elect), and the Western Network for Education in Health Services Administration (Chair). She is also a member of the American Public Health Association, American Association on Mental Retardation, Society on Disability Studies, and the International Association of Scientific Studies on Mental Deficiency.

Mary earned her M.H.A. in 1978 and her Ph.D. in educational psychology in 1984 from the University of Washington.